# walking with
# peety

# walking with
# peety

*The Dog Who Saved My Life*

# Eric O'Grey
## With Mark Dagostino

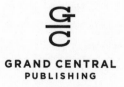

**GRAND CENTRAL**
**PUBLISHING**

NEW YORK   BOSTON

Copyright © 2017 by Eric O'Grey

Cover design by Elizabeth Connor.
Photograph of Peety courtesy of the author.
Photograph of grass © Gerald Bernard.
Cover copyright © 2017 by Hachette Book Group, Inc.

Grand Central Publishing
Hachette Book Group
1290 Avenue of the Americas, New York, NY 10104
grandcentralpublishing.com
twitter.com/grandcentralpub

First edition: October 2017

Grand Central Publishing is a division of Hachette Book Group, Inc. The Grand Central Publishing name and logo is a trademark of Hachette Book Group, Inc.

The publisher is not responsible for websites (or their content) that are not owned by the publisher.

The Hachette Speakers Bureau provides a wide range of authors for speaking events. To find out more, go to www.hachettespeakersbureau.com or call (866) 376-6591.

Library of Congress Cataloging-in-Publication Data has been applied for.

ISBNs: 978-1-4789-7116-0 (hardcover), 978-1-4789-7114-6 (ebook)

Printed in the United States of America

LSC-C

10  9  8  7  6  5  4  3  2  1

*To Peety,*

*I never knew what love was until you showed
me the true meaning of unconditional love.
I never knew what friendship was or cared
about anyone but myself until you showed me
the true meaning of selflessness.
I never knew what responsibility was until you
became responsible for me.
I am a better man in every aspect of my life
because of what you taught me.
Wait for me at the bridge on the riverbank. Be
a good boy and play in the grass and flowers,
and when you see me next we will cross the
bridge together into our next life.
I love you so much and will remember you
every day of my life.*

# contents

# Contents

# introduction

# Shadows and Light

When you're walking alone in a city late at night, the streetlights and glowing neon signs aren't all that comforting. All that brightness only makes the dark spots darker, casting deep shadows where unseen things can hide.

I suppose there are two ways to counter darkness: carry a big light wherever you go, or don't walk alone.

I never walked alone.

Peety was right there with me.

That scruffy old dog had taken me on a journey far greater than all of the road trips and adventures I'd managed to treat him to in the five years since we'd found each other. I was fully aware of how Peety had helped me to step onto my new path—the one I hoped to stay on for the rest of my life. I'd helped him step onto a new path, too, which is why it was tough to watch him that night. Even though his tail was wagging and he had that same bright look in his eye, I could tell he was walking a little slower than usual. I didn't think it was anything serious. To other people it probably looked like he was walking the way any healthy dog might walk. But from the moment we stepped out of our building I could tell he was struggling to keep up the regular pace we'd established over our many previous walks together.

I did the math in my head and realized we'd taken nearly two thousand walks since it all began. We'd walked a minimum of thirty minutes every morning, every evening, and lots of times in between, every day for all those years. That's a lot of paw prints on pavement.

Statistically, I knew the average life span of a medium-size dog is only ten to thirteen years. I also knew approximately how old Peety was, and I knew that those two numbers had converged. There was just no way I could believe that Peety was old enough to be slowing down, though. He was too joyful, too excited, too loving, and had way too much life in him for me to entertain the idea that he was in his so-called sunset years.

Plus, we were both too blissful to think morose thoughts. Since moving to Seattle, the two of us had been living like kings. Our downtown high-rise corner apartment had sweeping views over the lights of the city, the boats in Puget Sound, and even the Seahawks games down on Century-Link Field. From way up on the fourteenth floor, Peety could bark at every tiny dog he saw on the sidewalks below, just to let 'em know who was in charge.

Peety had his own balcony up there, complete with a private patch of sod, so he didn't have to wait to get fresh air or endure long elevator rides to go do his business. A crew of obedient humans showed up every two weeks to clean and replace his little patch of grass in the sky, as if he commanded his own court of loyal subjects.

It was *awesome*.

Best of all, he had a family. *We* had a family. My girlfriend Melissa and her kids loved Peety. They loved us both. I mean, what more could a dog want? (Or a man for that matter?) We were *happy*.

These are the things I kept telling myself while I tried to ignore his slower pace.

"Your dog is so adorable," an attractive young woman said as we turned the corner.

"Thank you," I replied. We kept on walking. Peety and I were used to that sort of attention. He *was* adorable with his patches of black-and-white fur, and knee-high stature. He'd been a babe magnet ever since he'd found his stride. A year or two earlier, I might have stopped and let that woman pet him. It would have made for a great introduction. But Peety and I were both much happier in the steady relationship we were in, that's for sure.

We decided to head east, away from the brightly lit, more touristy part of Pike Street, and were just about to cross Second Avenue when a panhandler stepped out of the darkness.

There are panhandlers all over downtown Seattle. Some are homeless. Some are college-age kids looking for drug money. Most are harmless. This guy wasn't. This guy was enormous, and intoxicated, and I could tell right away he was hell-bent on much more than borrowing a little spare change.

"You got money?" he said.

Peety stopped in his tracks, lowered his head, stared at the man, and growled.

"Sorry, man," I said. "Nothing on me. Come on, boy."

I tugged on his leash, but Peety wouldn't budge. He stood there, frozen. The hair on his neck stood up. His low, quiet growl grew deeper and louder.

"Ohhhh, what you think, that dog's gonna do something? That dog gonna hurt me?" The man raised his voice and stepped at me with a menacing look in his eye that made me stop in my tracks. Peety and I had walked this route a hundred times before without incident. I could not believe this was actually happening. Instinctively, my body tensed up, I squared my stance, and my fist gripped around Peety's leash, preparing to fight. I was strong, maybe stronger than I'd ever been. I'm pretty sure I could've handled myself in a fight. But this man was on something.

"Come on," he shouted. "I said give me some *money*!" He reached out to grab me, and Peety barked the most primal, vicious sound I'd ever heard. He jumped from the sidewalk—six full feet in the air—mouth open and lunging for the man's throat. I jerked on the leash and stopped him about an inch short of his teeth making contact. The panhandler reeled. He nearly fell over and scrambled on all fours before running back into the darkness.

Peety landed and tried to run after him, yanking on the leash, still barking, still holding his ground. I stared into the darkness right along with him, trying to see if the man was still there, trying to see whether he might be stupid enough to come back and face Peety's wrath.

Once I was convinced it was over, I looked at Peety—my

adorable boy—and I laughed. I couldn't help it. I could not understand where he found the strength and fearlessness to jump so high and protect me like that. He flew through the air like some kind of superdog! The only thing missing was a red cape and goggles.

As I looked back into the darkness, though, it hit me. I got tears in my eyes. I was positive that we had just come very close to the edge of something terrible. It was so unexpected. There had been no warning. Who knows what that man might have done to me? What if he had a knife, or a gun? I mean, that look in his eyes was something a person never wants to see. I took a deep breath and felt grateful that we were OK.

I felt as if I'd absentmindedly stepped off a curb in front of a speeding bus, only to have an angel grab my collar and pull me back from the brink.

I got down on one knee and petted the back of Peety's neck in long, calming strokes. "Good boy, Peety. Good boy, son," I said. "It's OK. It's OK now."

When Peety eased his stance, I stood back up. My voice broke when I said to him, "Let's go home."

Peety started walking again, only now, instead of walking at my side, he walked out in front of me—on patrol, guarding me like he had way back when this whole journey of ours first started.

I shook my head and wiped my cheeks on my sleeves.

I was sure that dog had just saved my life. For real. Which meant that Peety had now pretty much saved me in as many ways as a man could be saved.

Everywhere we went we would meet people who were

touched by the fact that I'd rescued Peety from an animal shelter. People seemed automatically impressed, as if that simple act of kindness somehow indicated that I was a good man. What I wanted to explain to every one of them was, "No. You've got it backward. This dog is the one who rescued *me*."

It felt odd to cut our walk short that night. We never cut our walks short. But I wanted to get home and tell Melissa what had happened.

She was just as thankful as I was that Peety had come to my rescue.

"What a good boy!" she said, dropping down to the floor to smother him with praise for his good deed. Peety let out a big sigh, as if his heroics were no big deal, but to me, watching those two cuddle was a big deal in and of itself. Melissa was deathly afraid of dogs before she met Peety. One of her kids was afraid of dogs, too.

My life was far from the only one Peety had changed, and I guess I should have known it was only the beginning.

It's funny. When you look back on moments like that—moments that you didn't realize were final moments at the time—they wind up holding more significance. But even then, that moment meant so much to me. When I looked in Peety's eyes, I knew that the two of us shared a bond as deep as any bond could be. So I smiled. And when Peety looked up at me from the warmth of Melissa's arms, he smiled right back at me. I couldn't help but fall down to my knees to hug him, too. That got him all riled up. He started licking my face so hard, he pushed me right over and climbed on top of my chest like a puppy. I laughed out loud, and that brought the kids running, and all of a sudden we all wound up in a big Peety pig-pile.

Man. Is there anything better than *that?*

That look in Peety's eyes. That trust. That protectiveness. That bond. That love. That unconditional love.

That's the thing that made all the difference in the world.

That's the thing that saved me—and I don't just mean from some angry panhandler.

That look is what saved me from myself.

# walking with
# peety

# chapter 1

## I'm Leaving . . .

*Traveling sucks.*

*Airports are the worst.*

*No, scratch that. Air*planes *are the worst.*

Oh, who am I kidding? Back then, it all sucked. Everything sucked. My work. My days. My nights. My *life*. I was miserable.

I was working in a job that wasn't exactly high on the list of dream jobs you envision when you're a kid. *Astronaut! Cowboy! Rock star! Movie star! Baseball player! Outside Salesman for a Major Appliance Company!* Yeah, no. And look, I'm not complaining. I was grateful just to have a job. I'd burned through dozens in the years leading up to that miserable day, and I'd lost one of them in such epic fashion that it required me to escape to the other side of the country. On a bus.

I hated buses, too. But back to the airport: any day I had to go to an airport was the worst day of my life. And this particular day quickly turned into the absolute worst of those very worst days.

Why is it that anywhere you park at the airport is a million-mile walk from where you need to be? I could feel myself tense up the moment I took my bag from the trunk of the rental car and stared at the stretched-out white lines marking the long walk in front of me. I was huffing and puffing before I was halfway to the door, and by the time I made it into the terminal my knees and ankles were pulsating. This despite the fact that I'd alternated doses of Tylenol and Advil every two hours from the moment I woke up just to prepare for the fact that I would have to walk that day at all.

On the escalator, some obnoxious kid (there was always some obnoxious kid) tried to hurry by me, only to find there wasn't enough room to pass. And instead of being patient, he tried to squish himself past me and the stainless-steel wall of the moving railing and nearly fell over, only to have his parents start yelling, "Tommy, stop! Don't do that! You're gonna get hurt! Say 'excuse me'! Oh, my gosh, I'm so sorry," as they and everyone around them looked in horror at the fat man who took up nearly the entire width of the moving staircase.

Yeah. That was me. I was *that* guy: the fat guy on his way home from a business trip, sweating through his button-down shirt and making everyone around him uncomfortable.

On this day in 2010, I weighed somewhere between 340 and 360 pounds. The exact number depended on whether you took my weight before or after one of my gargantuan-size meals, and depending on whose scale I stepped on. (The scale in the doctor's office always put me a good five or ten pounds heavier than I think I actually was. That happens to everyone, right? What's the deal with that? Are the laws of physics different in doctors' offices or something?)

I'm five-foot-ten, and my waist was fifty-two inches around. If you don't have a mental picture of that, picture this: my "love handles" were more like "hate pillows"— they rubbed against both sides of the metal detector as I squeezed my way through airport security.

The Transportation Security Administration (TSA) didn't provide benches in most airports back in 2010, and of course this was one of the airports that didn't have any benches available. Putting shoes back on from a standing position isn't a problem for most people. But I wasn't able to touch my feet, let alone tie my shoes, unless I was seated. And no, despite the well-meaning advice of others, loafers didn't make it easier. Slipping a loafer on required a tall shoehorn, and the TSA didn't provide those, either.

So I gathered my things and scuffed along the cold tile floor in my socks until I found a bench down the hall, and even then it took all my strength and will to compress my midsection enough to allow me to tie my shoes. That effort alone left me breathless. I had to stay on the bench for a good ten minutes afterward to rest.

When I stood up, the pain and numbness in my feet, legs, and knees radiated into my back. I looked at my boarding pass. I looked up at the gate numbers. I wanted to throw up. *Why is my gate always at the farthest end of the terminal?*

When I finally made it, there was no place to sit. The gate area was overflowing with passengers. Another full flight. We all realize we're getting ripped off, right? Treated like cattle? The luxurious side of the flight experience is all but gone.

Even skinny people realize that airline seats have become uncomfortably narrow. There wasn't a seat in the industry that could fit me without my fat spilling over into the seats on either side. If I were lucky enough to get a window or aisle seat, at least I would only press up against one other person. (Though, enduring the pain of the inevitable slam of the beverage cart was no fun for me, either.) I honestly needed two seats in order to fit my whole body, but my employer wasn't about to pay double for me to travel, and federal courts had ruled that obesity was not a "disability" within the meaning of the Americans with Disabilities Act. Therefore, neither the airlines nor my employer were required to provide any accommodations to alleviate the suffering of people in my condition.

On this day, on this oversold flight, I was assigned to a middle seat. Of course.

When my group number was called and I was forced to wait in yet another line to eventually board the plane, I leaned one shoulder against the wall of the Jetway in an attempt to alleviate the pressure on my knees. When I got to the plane, I realized it was one of the new models with a super-narrow aisle. I couldn't fit down the aisle facing forward. So I walked sideways, like a crab, watching the horrified faces of other passengers as I approached their rows. I could see their fear like cartoon thought bubbles above their heads: *"Please, God, don't let that humongous guy be in the seat next to me!"*

When I finally reached the unluckiest passengers on the plane—a generously sized white man on the aisle and a slender Korean man against the window—I said, "Pardon me. I'm in the center seat."

They didn't say anything. They didn't have to.

I wedged myself between the armrests of that seat knowing they would leave physical marks and possible bruising on my sides after the four-hour flight. Yet in my mind, I was sure that I was causing those two guys in my row more discomfort than I could possibly feel.

The seat belt wasn't long enough for me to buckle around my fifty-two-inch waist. They never were. So as always, I reached my right arm up, hoped desperately that my deodorant was still working, and hit the overhead call button to summon a flight attendant.

The nice lady looked and looked and, "Unfortunately," she said, there were several other large people on our flight that day, and the crew had "apparently" run out of seat belt extenders. I wasn't allowed to fly without one. They weren't allowed to take off unless all passengers were buckled in. So she hopped on that old-fashioned-looking phone handset on the cabin wall and called the gate to see if they had any extras.

They didn't. There were no extra seat belt extensions at the gate. To get one for me, they were going to have to transfer one from another plane.

"How long will this take?" the Korean man asked her.

"We'll take care of it as quickly as we can," the flight attendant said.

I thought I couldn't feel any worse than I already did. Then we sat there, waiting, and waiting. More than thirty minutes passed. Everyone was on board already, and everyone was getting upset. We were well past our departure time when the flight attendant finally came back and told me they'd located a seat belt extender and that we should be on our way shortly.

As soon as she left the Korean man said, quite loudly, "Great. I'm going to miss my connection because you're so fat!"

I wanted to die. Right there, in that seat, I wished my life would just end.

"I'm sorry," I said. I couldn't turn my giant neck around to actually look at him, and I wouldn't have had the strength to look him in the eye even if I could. I'd been morbidly obese for more than half my life at that point, and I'd learned it was easiest not to respond. It was better that way. So I just said one thing more: "I hope you have a pleasant flight."

The plane left the gate forty-five minutes late. As ridiculous as it sounds, I did my best to make myself small—to not be seen or heard or felt for the entire four-hour flight. I had to go to the bathroom, but I held it. I didn't want to make anyone move. I didn't want to make that walk.

When it was finally all over, I stepped back and let the Korean man exit the plane in front of me. He did so in a huff. I'm sure he missed his flight. I'm sure other people did, too. I'd single-handedly managed to inconvenience an entire plane full of people.

My sides hurt awful from the wedging of the armrests. Every joint in my body hurt as I made the long trek to my car. I collapsed into the driver's seat and nearly fell asleep in the parking garage from the sheer exhaustion of it all.

At home, I left my suitcase in the trunk. I couldn't bear the thought of carrying it all the way inside. I was starving. I collapsed on my couch and called Domino's. I ordered an extra-large meat-lover's pizza, and because it was the weekend, I ordered a second one to save for lunch the next day. (Less work.)

On that couch, I finished the first pizza. All of it. I was still hungry. "Just one more slice," I said to myself. Then after that slice went down, I ate another. And another. And another, till all that was left were two empty grease-stained boxes.

I ate both pizzas in one sitting.

An extra-large meat-lover's pizza is sixteen inches wide. It's not meant to be eaten by one person, or even two people. It's a party-size pizza. The ingredients in just one of them add up to somewhere around five thousand calories. That means I consumed around ten thousand calories in a single sitting. Not that I knew these nutrition facts at the time. I didn't pay attention to those sorts of things. I was hungry, so I ate.

Oh, and that two-extra-large-pizzas-in-one-sitting thing? It wasn't my first time. In fact, it had become my Friday-night routine. I always said I would eat one and save one. I always wound up eating them both. It was one of a million routines that made me feel ashamed and depressed every time it happened—but I didn't know how to stop. I didn't understand what was wrong with me. I beat myself up over everything I did. I didn't know how to get better.

I'd already spent twenty-five years trying every diet and diet product I'd ever seen advertised on TV and in magazines. I'd even tried some not-commercially-available diet products that nearly did me in. Not a single one of them had worked. Sure, I dropped some weight at first. I dropped a good forty pounds using some of those gimmicks and fad diets, and I felt better for a few weeks, or even a few months. But eventually, I would cheat. I'd get sick of the lousy prepackaged food. I'd miss a meeting. Whatever it was, I would backslide. I'd feel miserable after doing that, and then I'd just give up. The diet would end and I'd go right back to my Standard American Diet of greasy fast food and home delivery.

In a matter of weeks, the weight always came back—and then some.

I know I'm not alone in this. I know half of America has had the same experience. I just did it to the extreme.

When I was finally done eating that night of the terrible flight, I got up to go to bed. That's when I caught a glimpse of the pile of dirty underwear in the spare bedroom, and I realized just how broken I really was.

My discarded underwear had piled up high enough that I could see the top of the mound over the edge of the spare bed. I did the math in my head and estimated there was more than a thousand pairs in there. I had given up on doing laundry long ago. It was just too big of an ordeal to get to the coin washers in my building. So I had a cleaning service pick up and deliver my laundry instead, and rather than go through the hassle of washing and reusing my underwear, I decided to order new underwear and socks every few weeks from Amazon. I had new ones delivered to my door, just like my pizzas. I threw the dirty ones in the spare bedroom, where I couldn't see them, and where I knew no one else would see them, either.

No one ever came to my apartment. I'd stopped going

to other people's homes, too. I had basically given up on maintaining any friendships at all. It was just too much for me. Everything outside of my apartment was too much for me. I'd set myself up so I could do most of my work from home, on the phone and on the computer. Personal sales calls and business travel were just about the only reasons I ever stepped foot into the outside world, and I only did that because I had to.

About a year before then, I'd dragged myself to a company-mandated physical, where after looking at my blood work the doctor strongly suggested that I buy a cemetery plot.

"What?" I said.

"If you don't get your weight under control, you're going to need one in the next five years."

*Who does he think he is?* I thought. I was angry at him for being so rude. I walked out vowing to find another doctor.

Still, a blunt doctor's words can be powerful. I absolutely took his words to heart. But not in a good way. Not in a motivational way. In more of a fatalistic way.

It struck me that night that I'd already blown through one fifth of the life I had left. Nothing had gotten better in that year. In fact, everything was worse. *Everything.*

I hadn't been on a date in fifteen years. The pile of underwear looked like something out of a movie, like something some person who had lost his mind had piled up while they turned into a recluse and slipped away from reality.

Is that what I was now? A crazy person? A recluse?

*How did I let this happen?*

I had type 2 diabetes, and it was out of control. I had

read all the warnings. I knew that if I didn't get it under control, I'd go blind or lose a limb. And yet nothing I did seemed to help. Part of the reason I had to work so hard was to earn enough money to pay for my medication. Even with insurance, it cost me up to a thousand dollars in co-payments every month for the prescription medications I needed just to survive. I needed medicine to help with my insulin levels, and to fight my high blood pressure and deadly cholesterol levels. I needed more prescriptions to help me sleep, prescriptions for anxiety and depression, and even more medications just to counter the side effects of the other medications. And none of them made me feel better. None of them. I felt miserable. All the time.

The blunt doctor referred me to a bariatric surgeon—a guy who wanted to cut me open and remove a large portion of my stomach just to get my eating under control. The surgery sounded barbaric to me. And yet, I had gone through the whole pre-prep process and told them to go ahead and schedule me in. It was scheduled to happen a month from that very day. That's how desperate I was.

I didn't want that surgery. I couldn't do that to my body. It seemed grotesque. How could I allow someone to cut out my insides to try to stop something that was all my fault in the first place? *How did this all happen? Why can't I stop eating? Are they really going to cut me open and remove part of my stomach?*

I couldn't do that. I wouldn't.

*No.*

I knew what I wanted. I knew what needed to happen. I didn't own a gun. I wasn't taking any pills that seemed strong enough to do the job. Perhaps I could just stand in front of a train. I didn't know how to do it, but after the day I'd had, I knew it had to be done. I just wished I had followed my doctor's advice and gone ahead and purchased a plot at the local cemetery.

*I didn't even do that right*, I thought.

Every single part of my body ached in flu-like pain as I collapsed into bed. My stomach churned from all the grease and fat and cheese. The physical agony of it was more than I could take. I turned off the light, and with tears in my eyes I did something I had never done before.

I prayed.

"God," I said into the darkness of my room, "I'm begging you. Please kill me. Please take my life. Please."

# chapter 2

## Waking Up

What happened next might sound strange to some people. Heck, it still sounds strange to me.

I didn't die.

Instead, after praying for my life to be taken, I blacked out.

Some might call it a dream, some might call it a delusion, but I found myself being pulled into a vortex of white light. It felt like I was falling and flying all at the same time, but it wasn't scary. It was peaceful. I didn't see a divine being or the pearly gates of heaven, and there wasn't even a booming voice. In fact, in this dream (or whatever it was) there were no words spoken at all. All I knew is I suddenly felt full of hope—and I was positive I was no longer alone. I was in the presence of God.

I'd never gone to church in my life other than for weddings and funerals. I wasn't raised with any religion. The fact that I'd prayed to God in my moment of desperation came as a complete surprise to me. And yet, God is what I felt.

I understand there are those who will think this next part sounds crazy, too. Before it happened to me, I might have thought it was crazy myself. But I slept through the night and woke up in the morning feeling empowered. Even though it was a Saturday, and I would normally have spent most of my weekend in bed, I got up. I showered. I got dressed. I took the elevator down and stepped out onto the sidewalk. I felt the warmth of the sun on my face and noticed the green of the palm trees. I noticed the ridge of snow-capped mountains in the distance through the hazy San Jose sky. I then rode the elevator back up to my apartment, stepped inside, picked up my laptop, and ordered a Bible from Amazon. I can't explain why I did that. I just knew it was something I had to do.

Two days later, a Bible showed up at my front door, just as with a pizza, I devoured it. I spent every free hour for the better part of next month reading every word of that New Living Translation Life Application Study Bible, cover to cover. I don't remember doing anything else with my life that month besides reading those words. My body still ached. I still felt miserable. But I felt like I was on a mission to finish that book. So I only worked as much as I had to. I turned off the TV. I ate steady rations of pizza, Chinese delivery, and fast food from the nearest drive-throughs. And I read.

There were parts of the Bible that made no sense to me and parts that resonated deeply—as if they'd been written just for me. I encountered dozens and dozens of stories I'd never heard before, and I recognized many common phrases, sayings, and references that people use in their daily lives that I'd never realized were drawn from the Bible. I read all

of the historical references in the footnotes and was flabber-
gasted to discover how many events in the Bible lined up
with the non-religious history I'd learned in school. I was
an avid reader of all sorts of books, and I simply could not
believe I had gone through fifty-one years of life without
reading or even attempting to understand the power that so
many people found in those pages.

When I finally reached the end of the final sentence of
Revelation, I was sitting on my couch. I closed the book with
a sense of satisfaction, as if I had done a good thing—and
suddenly, once again, I blacked out. I found myself drawn
into that same bright vortex. Again no words were spoken;
yet I heard a message loud and clear. The beautiful and ra-
diant presence told me not to despair. He asked me (without
words) to repent my sins, to give myself to Him, and to trust
Him with my life.

Perhaps because I had nothing left to lose, I said, "Yes."

And then He told me that I should never fear again, because I was sealed from evil and protected from harm until
the end of my days, and that I should go forth in peace, follow the signs I would receive, and wait for my purpose to be
revealed.

I woke up sprawled on my living room floor.

I have no memory of how I got there.

I have no idea how long I was out.

The morning sun came streaming through the blinds,
and it was unlike any light I had ever seen. I can only describe it as if the light were streaming through the ornate
stained glass of some European cathedral, in a beautifully
shot film, in hues of yellow and gold. My whole apartment

seemed to glow. Every object lit up. I looked around from my beached-whale position on the floor and felt like I was seeing everything in that room for the very first time. It was strange, and beautiful. But the thing I remember most is the overwhelming feeling I had—a feeling that was the exact opposite of what I'd felt when I prayed through tears.

I no longer wanted to die.

Instead, I wanted to *live*.

What anyone else wants to call my experience is up to them. The few people I dared to tell about these experiences suggested that maybe they were a medical event, that perhaps I'd suffered a series of heart attacks or minor strokes. I don't think that's the case, but I also don't think it matters. Any way I look at it, it felt to me like a divine intervention.

I had hit rock bottom. The kind of "rock bottom" you usually hear about from alcoholics and drug addicts.

I woke up from a very dark place knowing that I wanted to live, and I woke up knowing that in order to live, I needed to change.

I felt motivated for the first time in decades. Motivated to do *what*, I wasn't sure. I'd already exhausted every diet under the sun in my previous attempts to get my life back. But there was something different about the motivation I felt this time. I felt that I was seeing things in an entirely new way, and that my desire to live now outshined any obstacle that might get in my way.

I opened my eyes and started actively looking for signs that might lead me toward a better life—and immediately a sign showed up.

After I managed to roll myself over and achingly lift myself from the floor to the couch, I turned on the TV. And while I caught my breath, I just happened to catch Wolf Blitzer in the middle of an interview with former president Bill Clinton. (I can assure you, those are not two people from whom I expected to receive a sign.)

Wolf said something to the former president about how great he looked—and I had to admit, he looked pretty great. I remembered seeing pictures of Mr. Clinton at the end of his eight years looking beleaguered, old, tired, and kind of bloated. Now here he was on CNN looking fit and full of energy. He truly looked about half his former size. It was stunning. His face was oval instead of round, and the heavy bags under his eyes were gone. He looked like a whole new person. When Wolf asked him how he'd done it, Mr. Clinton said that he'd been under the care of a doctor who put him on a whole-food, plant-based diet. That was all it took, he said, to completely change the way he felt. He lost weight without feeling hungry, and he was healthier and stronger than he'd been since his twenties.

I had no idea what a "whole-food, plant-based diet" was, but I took it as the sign I was looking for and ran with it. I didn't actually "run," of course. I couldn't run to save my life. But I managed to lean my girth over to my travel bag and pull out my laptop. I went online and searched for "plant-based diets" and came up with a few names right in my local area. It wasn't hard: I lived in San Jose, California, in the Silicon Valley region just south of San Francisco. There was no shortage of nutritionists and other health gurus available. But before that moment, I had never shown any interest in any of that Left-Coast, Yoga-loving, new-age mumbo jumbo (as I might have referred to it back then). I was raised in the area, sure, but I wasn't raised by hippies. I'd joined the army immediately after high school. I'd spent several years in Atlanta, Georgia, eating fried chicken and peach cobbler, sometimes both, for breakfast. That whole San Francisco tree-hugging, save-the-world, healthy-mind/healthy-body mentality never held any appeal for me.

Still, I could not shake the overwhelming feeling that I needed to follow whatever signs showed up.

I wasn't an idiot about it. I didn't go about it blindly. I was (and still am) a good salesman, and I'd been an attorney once, so I knew how to do research. I also knew I didn't want to try anything that was just another fad diet. I didn't want to do anything gimmicky that might risk making my health worse than it already was. So I made a conscious effort to find an actual doctor—someone who was certified and had all of the degrees that a "real" doctor would have—but who was trained in nutrition and knowledgeable about the plant-based diet that Bill Clinton had talked about on TV.

Within an hour I had found a couple of naturopathic doctors who seemed legit. I called them. I asked if they could see me right away, and of course they couldn't. I don't think nutritionists are in the habit of receiving emergency calls, and despite my desperate pleas, they offered to book me an introductory appointment a month or two down the road. I knew I couldn't wait that long. My need to tackle this felt like a fire inside of me now. I honestly felt like I might not stay alive if I put it off for another day. So I kept trying.

Finally, I came across Dr. Preeti Kulkarni, a woman with

the qualifications I was looking for who also had wonderful reviews from a long list of patients. I got through to her office, told her my situation, and she agreed to see me the very next day. It felt like this was meant to be.

It also felt as if I were still floating in the afterglow in my car on the way to her office. The whole world seemed somehow brighter. That feeling that I wanted to live, and I mean really *live*—to finally put an end to my misery, once and for all—would not go away. So as I drove, I resolved myself to try something new: I decided I was going to do whatever this woman told me to do. I wasn't going to second-guess her. I wasn't going to take just some of her advice and then do my own thing because I "knew better" or even "knew myself better." It was very clear to me that I *didn't* know better. I'd been down the diet road dozens of times before that moment. I'd tried to fix myself and failed miserably. I recalled a phrase I'd heard somewhere—"The definition of insanity is doing the same thing over and over again and expecting different results"—and I knew in my heart that the only way this effort would possibly yield different results was if I did things differently. *Really* differently. So I resolved to follow this doctor's instructions, strictly. I would do everything she told me to do.

If it still didn't work? Well, then, that was that.

Dr. Preeti (as she liked to be called) was younger than I expected. I guess we all feel that way in middle age, when our doctors look as though they could be our grown children. It feels somehow wrong, as if the world is upside down. But in this case, it felt perfect. It was different for me, and different was good. She was also tiny in stature, which exacerbated how young she looked. *She would definitely be carded if she tried to buy a bottle of wine,* I thought. She barely came up to my chest. But there was something reassuring about her the moment we met. She had a calmness that made her seem entirely focused and professional. She looked me in the eye with the sort of easygoing confidence of someone who knows exactly what they're doing.

And she didn't seem repulsed by my weight.

My eye contact didn't last long, though. It never did. As soon as we sat down in her office I could feel my eyes bore into the industrial-gray carpet near her sensible shoes.

"So, tell me about yourself," she said. "Are you married? Single?"

"I'm single," I said.

"Dating?"

"Umm, no. Not for many years."

*Dating?* I'd never had a doctor ask me if I was dating before. I thought it was a really odd thing to ask.

"Well, what do you like to do for fun?"

I looked up at her face just to make sure I was still in the right office.

"I…ummm…well, I like to read, I guess."

"Any social activities?"

"No. Not really."

She kept on like this for a good half hour. She wanted to know where I lived, and what I did for work, and if I'd ever played any sports.

I finally stopped and asked her, "Why are you asking all of this? I mean, I don't think I've ever had a doctor spend more than ten minutes with me before giving me a prescription and sending me on my way."

"Yes, so, I know the reason you called me, and you want help losing weight, and what I like to tell my patients is this isn't about losing weight. Diets and 'losing weight' for the sake of losing weight don't really work, right? I assume you've tried dieting?"

"Yeah, of course. I've tried every diet there is."

"Right. A lot of my patients say that. And we should go over those diets, just so I know what you've tried. But what I want is for you to get healthy, so that your body starts working for you instead of against you. And so what I do, and what all naturopathic doctors do, is not to try to treat the symptoms you have—which, your weight is really a symptom—but instead to treat *you*, the whole person, to get to the root cause of any ailment you might have, including your weight. Does that make sense?"

"Yeah," I said. "Yeah. That actually makes a lot of sense."

"So," she said, "now that I know a little bit about you, why don't you go ahead and tell me about your diet."

"Well, I'm not on any diet right now."

"No, I mean, what do you eat on a daily basis. Do you like to cook?"

"Ha!" I laughed.

"What's so funny?"

"I'm an appliance salesman who never turns on his own stove."

"Never? You must cook sometimes."

"I can boil water, so I make instant Ramen once in a while. Does that count?" She wasn't much for laughing, it seemed. "I have made a grilled cheese sandwich a few times."

"So, where do you get most of your food, then?"

"Delivery mostly," I said. I told her about the pizzas. She took notes. "I also just go to drive-throughs, so I don't have to get out of the car."

"So, McDonald's? Fast food? What do you order?"

"Yeah. For breakfast I'll get five or six Egg McMuffins. Lunch, usually three or four Big Macs and a couple of large fries."

"How about anywhere else? Any fruits or vegetables?"

"Orange juice, sometimes. But no. I'm not really a veggie eater."

"OK, and on your Egg McMuffins, are those with bacon, ham—"

"Yes."

"Always meat?"

"Yeah, for sure."

"Cheese?"

"Yup."

"Do you drink a lot of milk?"

"No. I gave up milk when I was a kid. I had bad acne and I noticed it went away when I stopped drinking milk."

"Oh. That's good. Are there other changes you've noticed when you gave up certain foods?"

I thought about it, and I couldn't think of a single food I'd given up in all the years since. The idea of how easy it was to give up a food as a way to change something I didn't like on my body hadn't really occurred to me since I was a teenager.

By the end of our visit, it's safe to say that Dr. Preeti knew a lot about my life and habits. She set me up to go get some blood work done and a whole battery of tests to assess my "overall health," she said. Then she spoke to me about her expectations for what would happen if I switched to a whole-food, plant-based diet under her guidance.

"The reason I'll be testing your adrenals and doing the blood work is to look for nutritional deficiencies. If you're deficient in certain nutrients, it's hard to get back into health without correcting that. So we might start with some supplements to kick-start your system and get things back into balance. But by switching to a plant-based diet, once your nutritional needs are met, and your digestion is optimum, you won't need meds or supplements to stay healthy," she said.

I reminded her that I had type 2 diabetes, high cholesterol, high blood pressure. I was on all sorts of meds for those.

"Now, yes. But if you stick to what I tell you, there's a good chance you won't need any of those in a few months."

"Are you saying everything that's wrong with me can be treated just by switching what I eat, and, like, counting calories and stuff?"

"Yes and no. What I'm saying is our bodies need nutrition and energy, and what you're feeding your body matters. It matters more than most people know. Even for people who sometimes think they're 'healthy.' But it's not complicated. I promise. You can forget about counting calories for now. To get started, at every meal, just make sure that at least half your plate is full of fruits and vegetables and the rest is beans and rice or any other food that is not from an animal," she said. "If you do that, you'll start feeling better. And with exercise, I think you'll really be surprised how quickly things can change."

"Exercise?" I said.

I knew that last part was going to be my undoing. I didn't have the strength or energy to do any sort of exercise. I had *tried*. I had wasted so much money on gym memberships over the years, and I knew I was too old to change my ways now. I hated going to the gym. I hated the smell of it, the agony of it, the pain of those tiny, hard, sticky rubber seats on the bike machines. I hated the stigma of standing without clothes on in a locker room, feeling the stares and whispers behind my back. I was still resolved to do whatever she told me, but I knew that if she required me to make trips to the gym, then this whole endeavor would be really short-lived.

"What I recommend to start is just twenty minutes of light exercise, twice a day. Something you can enjoy, like taking a walk," she said.

*If you think I enjoy taking walks, then you haven't listened to a word I said,* I thought.

"And in your case, I recommend that you go to a shelter and adopt a dog," she added.

Once again, her words caused me to raise my stare from the floor.

"A dog?"

"Yes. A dog is a good companion. I think it will be beneficial for you to have a companion. Plus, you live in an apartment, which means the dog has to be walked. So you walk your dog twice a day, and that will be your exercise. Easy."

"I've never owned a dog. What about a cat?" I asked.

"Have you ever seen anyone walk a cat?"

"I think I did on TV once," I said.

She looked at me sternly.

I felt foolish.

"A cat is a nice companion, but really, go to the shelter. I just read an article about the Humane Society here in Silicon Valley. There are so many dogs there that need to be adopted. It will give you something to focus on, a partner to take care of and hopefully bond with, and, believe me, that dog will get you up and moving and out of your apartment. It will help in ways you haven't even begun to think about, too."

How could I take care of a dog? I'd never owned a pet in my life. I started to imagine what a hassle it would be: having to buy pet food, having to bend over all the way to the ground to pick up dog poop.

Plus, I had to travel on business. What would I do with a dog? I was sure I wasn't a "dog person."

But then I remembered my resolution in the car: *do whatever this woman says*.

Dr. Preeti had spent more than an hour and a half with me on my very first visit. I was shell shocked and wondered if I'd be able to remember everything she said.

On the way out, she insisted I sign up and pre-pay for six months of weekly appointments in her office, because that would make me commit to follow this program. Fortunately, my insurance co-pay was only twenty-five dollars per visit. But it worked. If I wasn't fully committed before, I felt financially committed now. She then handed me a big printout of recipes and a list of ingredients for vegetarian dishes and meals and healthy snacks that I should go buy. I couldn't help but think, *I hate vegetables*, and yet I kept coming back to my resolution: *just do what she says*. She told me she would be much more specific about what foods to eat once my blood work came back, but in the meantime she asked that I try as hard as I could to stop eating any meat or dairy products. She said the best way to do that might be to ration it out: "Give yourself an allowance of six cans of tuna for the next two weeks, for instance, and only eat them when you really, really crave it. Then once they're gone, they are gone," she said.

I nodded and agreed to all of it. I felt dazed.

"And I really do hope you go pick out a dog. It's a big commitment, but you won't regret it," she said. "Take care now, Eric. It was very nice to meet you."

I looked her in the eyes and I said, "OK."

# chapter 3

# The Perfect Pup

I could feel my heart pounding in my chest. I could feel my knees throbbing, too, but I was pretty sure the walk from Dr. Preeti's office to my car wasn't the cause of my rapid heart rate. As I sat there in the parking lot flipping through the long list of alleged "meals" she wanted me to prepare for myself, I realized I couldn't do it.

*I hate vegetables.*

*I can't cook.*

*Rice and beans? That's not a meal. That's a side dish!*

*What the hell was I thinking?*

I racked my brain trying to think of even one meal in my entire life that didn't include some sort of meat, or cheese, or other "animal product." Yeah. She didn't want me to eat meat, dairy, or *animal products.* It suddenly dawned on me that this whole-food, plant-based diet thing was actually the "vegan" diet I'd heard about over the years.

*This is what hippies eat. Is she asking me to become a hippie?*

I'd met a few vegans. I lived in the San Francisco Bay

Area, near places like Santa Cruz and Berkeley, where people sang "Kumbaya" in parks and wore purple hair and Birkenstock sandals with different-colored socks. These people seemed like the most extreme version of vegetarian, animal-rights activists I'd ever encountered. They seemed nothing like me, and I thought I had nothing in common with them.

Then again, Dr. Preeti said she practiced this diet herself, and she certainly didn't seem like a hippie, so that gave me some hope that maybe my opinion of all vegans wasn't exactly accurate. But the list of things I couldn't eat on this diet seemed ridiculously long.

*She doesn't want me to eat eggs? No eggs? What the hell am I supposed to eat for breakfast?*

I nearly laughed out loud at how ridiculous it all seemed.

*And me with a dog?* I thought about the vet bills. The dog food. *What on earth will I do when I go on business trips? My apartment will be covered in dog hair. I'll have hair all over my business clothes. What if it takes a poop on the floor? I certainly don't want to have to clean that up myself. What does she expect me to do, hire someone to clean my apartment? This might be the most expensive diet I've ever tried!*

I'd gone into that appointment feeling positive that I could follow this doctor's orders. I'd convinced myself that this was my very last shot. Yet I could not understand how any of this was possibly going to work for me.

I tossed the printout on the passenger seat and gripped the steering wheel. I stared at the brick wall in front of me.

I quickly realized I was doing what I always did: getting discouraged. Panicking. I was angry at myself for allowing myself to get this way, and mad that I was already expressing that anger by blaming my life on another diet that was impossible to follow.

The fact is, I knew deep down that this really was my last shot.

And suddenly I remembered something I'd read in the Bible.

> *Trust in the Lord with all your heart; do not*
> *depend on your own understanding.*
> —Proverbs 3:5 (NLT)

I closed my eyes and tried to breathe. I tried to recall and embrace that awesome, powerfully positive feeling I'd experienced in my apartment when I woke up on the floor in the glow of the streaming sun. I tried to trust that I was following the signs God had shown me (as extraordinary as that still seemed to me on its face).

*I have to at least try*, I thought. *Don't give up yet.*

I started the car and made up my mind to drive to Safeway, even though I hated grocery stores. Walking up and down those long aisles was almost as excruciating as a trip to the airport. The Safeway near my apartment was nothing special, as far as supermarkets go, but at least it had wide aisles. There were some smaller grocery stores I'd shopped where my body would block anyone else from getting by in the aisles, causing dozens of awkward, side-turning, squeeze-by moments or forcing me to back my cart up like a bus on a one-way street so other people could pass. That would happen dozens of times in a single trip. Not to mention the stares I'd get from some obnoxious kid, or the look of revulsion from some thin-as-a-rail nineteen-year-old California girl. It was exhausting and humiliating—and not exactly how a person wants to feel while spending money.

I'd given up on buying fresh produce a decade or so earlier, anyway. All it ever did was rot in the bottom drawer of my refrigerator. I'd always wind up throwing away those thin, clear, plastic bags full of brown, soupy, moldy blobs a few months later. So why bother? Why on earth would anyone purchase anything other than canned, frozen, or packaged foods with at least a six-month expiration date? And really, why even go to the grocery store? Non-perishable items could be bought online and delivered, just like my underwear and everything else. For meals, it was easier to follow the "window diet"—eating whatever could be handed to me through the window of my car or the front door of my apartment. The less human interaction the better.

I knew I didn't have a single ingredient on Dr. Preeti's list in my apartment, though. So if I wanted to try to get this started, I simply had to do this.

No sooner did I pull out of the parking lot than I saw a woman in yoga pants walking a Chihuahua at the end of a pink, crystal-studded leash. The dog looked like a little rat to me. I was definitely not going to become the owner of one of those. Then two blocks down I saw another woman walking another dog, a big brown dog of some sort that came up to her waist, and all I could think about was what a pain it would be to deal with that size dog in my apartment.

I saw another dog, a Labrador retriever, tied to a signpost just outside the Safeway, anxiously awaiting its owner, and a poodle of some kind panting like crazy in the backseat of the car next to mine when I parked. Suddenly there were dogs everywhere. I was surrounded by them! It was weird. I had never seen that many dogs in my neighborhood, ever.

My ankles hurt as I grabbed a shopping cart and lumbered inside with the ingredient list in hand. I followed the flow of human traffic through the entire dairy section, realizing there wasn't a single thing on my list in that whole section. I passed the deli counter in the back as I looked at the signs above the aisles, hoping to find any sign of the foreign-sounding ingredients I supposedly needed.

*What the hell is "quinoa"? And how the hell do I pronounce it?*

I finally saw a single aisle that held two of the most-repeated ingredients: rice and beans. I hadn't really spent any time in that aisle before, so I was completely clueless about how to make sense of it all. There were boxes of rice, and instant bags of rice, little cups of rice made for micro-waving, Spanish rice, Basmati rice, wild rice, rice blends, until finally I saw a big clear bag of something called long-grain brown rice. *That sounds right.* I threw it in the cart.

The beans were even more baffling. I had no idea what to get or how to cook them. I flipped one bag over and it said the beans needed to be soaked for eight hours before cook-ing. *Eight hours? I don't have eight hours. I need these for dinner.* So I looked at the canned beans and picked out some red ones and black ones and threw them in the cart.

Just then, a young woman came walking up the aisle with a black-haired, toddler-aged girl perched in the front of her cart. Not on the seat, but up in the main part of the cart where she could walk around, like she was in a little cage at the zoo, only on wheels. The toddler was sort of singing to herself and swaying her pale yellow dress back and forth to some music in her head. Then she stood at the very front of the cart and put her arms up in the air, like she was Kate Winslet on the bow of the Titanic, all "King of the World"–style as she floated past the garbanzo beans. All of a sudden she opened her eyes and saw me, and she gasped. She looked scared. Then she laughed. She turned around quickly and said, "Look, Mommy! A giant!"

Her mommy said, "Ay!" and started whisper-shouting at the little girl in Spanish. "I'm so sorry," she said as she scooted by me at a quicker pace.

"It's all right," I said, even though it really wasn't.

I was already tired, and now I felt like crawling into a cave. I decided to take the quickest route possible to get out of there. I thought about Dr. Preeti's advice: at least *half of your plate should be fresh fruits and vegetables*. Since there were no fruits and vegetables anywhere in the center aisles of the grocery store, I beelined it to the produce section. Again, I didn't recognize the names of many of the fruits and vegetables listed on her pages, so I decided to keep it simple. I picked up some oranges. I picked up some apples. I grabbed a bunch of bananas. I knew I didn't like broccoli, but I heard the echoes of my mother in my head, saying *"How do you know you don't like it if you have never even tried it?"* Then I thought, *Never mind, my mother didn't like vegetables, either.* I grew up in the '60s, when everyone I knew pretty much ate everything out of boxes and cans. But I resigned myself to my new fate and threw a big head of broccoli into my cart.

Before I left, I grabbed a loaf of bread, too. I figured I'd have some toast for breakfast in the morning. That and coffee had gotten me out the door of many a hotel over the years. The good old continental breakfast. I figured it ought to work just as well now. I was pretty sure I had butter and jelly in my fridge (although, there was no telling how old it was).

I also grabbed my allowance of six cans of tuna. My non-vegetarian outs. My backup plan to help wean me away from my current diet.

As I went through the checkout line, I noticed the cashier taking a longer-than-normal look at my stomach. I looked down and saw a big black line of a stain across the widest part of my shirt, right above my belly button and stretching off to the right. It must have come from one of the produce cases, probably when I was forced to squish against it while reaching for the ripe bananas at the top of the pile.

The cashier didn't say anything, but I knew what she was thinking.

I looked like a slob. A big fat giant slob. One more humiliation.

In the parking lot, I found myself gripping the steering wheel again, trying again not to lose my composure. Trying to move forward.

I went home, lugged my haul to my apartment, put it all away, and collapsed on the couch.

When I woke from my midafternoon nap, I made a few phone calls for work before turning my attention to the next task at hand: trying to wrap my head around getting a dog.

I Googled "adopt a dog San Jose," and all sorts of things

popped up. There were independent dog rescue centers, links steering me to People for the Ethical Treatment of Animals (PETA) and the American Society for the Prevention of Cruelty to Animals (ASPCA), and pet stores, but the one that jumped out at me right away was Humane Society Silicon Valley (HSSV)—the organization Dr. Preeti had mentioned. They had, by far, the largest selection of adoptable dogs listed on their site, so I just started browsing.

They had perfect little eight-pound poodles that were really cute. One was named Fifi. I could picture her walking along, prancing like a Kentucky horse in a pink-studded collar. *Not for me*, I thought. It seemed like they had a lot of Chihuahuas. And so many other breeds! There were brown dogs, black ones, tan ones, white ones, spotted ones, ones with short hair, long hair, and mixes. And who knew that a Chihuahua could mate with a pit bull? What would you even call that combination? A pithuahua or a chibull? I loved the look of pit bulls; they were "manly" dogs for sure. But I kept scrolling and found a whole range of dogs in between, with detailed descriptions and disclaimers. One said, "No cats or small children," and another said, "Perfect for families with small children: rated E for everyone!"

I was back in the mind-set of really wanting to make this work, so I started Googling the various characteristics of different breeds, and thinking about the ideal dog for me: one that would be a joy and delight from the start, would be happy, wouldn't have any attitude problems, would never, ever pee or poop inside (not one time ever in the history of the dog), would never bark, would always be quiet, wouldn't shed, and would definitely never, ever pull down my curtains, chew on my furniture, or eat my shoes. By the end of all of my research, I was finally able to visualize my ideal dog: a happy, pretrained, fully grown eight-pound golden retriever.

Even though it was near the end of the day, I decided not to wait. I called the HSSV number and told the nice lady who answered exactly what I was looking for.

"Do you have any dogs like that?" I asked.

"Ummm..." the young lady said. "Let me put you through to Casaundra. She handles our fosters and adoptions, and she can walk you through the process. Please hold."

Not a minute later, I began the conversation that would forever change my life.

"This is Casaundra. Is this Eric?"

"It is."

"I hear you're looking to adopt a dog."

"Yes. Well, my doctor basically prescribed a dog for me, and said I should go to the shelter and adopt one, and I've never owned a dog before, so I'm looking for a dog that will be really easy to care for, friendly, gets along with everyone, isn't too big, doesn't shed, won't bark or disturb my neighbors, and won't pee or poop in my apartment. I don't know what breed that would be, but I have this picture in my head, and I'm just hoping you might have a dog that fits that description," I said, pretty much all in one breath.

"Your doctor prescribed you a dog?"

"She did. She's a naturopathic doctor, and she believes in

holistic medicine and treating the whole person. And, well, she really thinks a dog will be good for me."

"Oh. For what reason?"

"Everything, really. I guess I should tell you that I'm overweight. A lot overweight. But I'm trying to change that. So she's putting me on a new diet, and one of the reasons she wants me to have a dog is so I'll go outside and get some exercise by walking him twice a day."

"Oh," Casaundra said. "Well, what I'd like to do is ask you a few questions, and hopefully that will give me a better understanding of what you're looking for, and what you might be able to offer to one of our animals."

*Offer to one of her animals?*

"OK, sure," I said.

For the next forty minutes, Casaundra grilled me. She asked me almost as many questions about my life and background and intentions for this imaginary dog I envisioned as Dr. Preeti had asked me about myself that morning. From, "Do you live alone?" to "Have you ever owned a pet of any kind?" to "How much walking do you do now?"

"Well, I haven't started yet," I admitted. "But I plan to start right away."

I remember thinking, *Wow. This is a lot of work to adopt a dog. I thought I'd just tell them what kind I want and go pick it up, or maybe they could deliver it!*

She asked me whether I had friends with dogs, and how I reacted to dogs at friends' houses, and in public, and about what kind of a job I had, and how much I traveled.

Throughout the phone call she also kept circling back to the idea of this being a "lifetime commitment."

"A dog isn't a toy. You can't just do a trial run and give up. They need love and attention, and they bond with their families, you know? They want to be part of a family. Are you committed to this idea? Can you stay committed?"

From the tone in her voice, I could tell this was extremely important to her. It really mattered. So I thought about it for a few seconds, and my answer was clear: "Yeah," I said. "I'm truly going to give my all to this. It's important to me that I see this through. In a lot of ways, I think my life depends on it. But I understand why you're asking. It's a big commitment for sure. I mean, maybe I should get an older dog so the commitment isn't as long. Would that be easier?"

(Looking back on it now, I still can't believe I asked that question. I honestly thought, *An older dog will only live a couple of years, which would be a shorter commitment.* Man, would I come to regret that way of thinking.)

"I don't know about that," Casaundra said.

"All I know is that I want this to work. It'll be an adjustment for me, and I'm nervous about that. But everything in me is telling me to follow this doctor's advice. I went to the supermarket right after I left her office, and I bought rice and beans for dinner, because I'm dead-set on losing weight and getting healthy. I want to live. I want to change my life for the better. I really do," I said, "and Dr. Preeti really seems to think that a dog will help me with that."

Casaundra was definitely a good listener. As a salesman, I always try to ask my customers lots of questions. I want to find out everything I can about them so I can sell them the product that best suits them. If they're happy with the sale, they will come back to me the next time, and the next, and recommend me to their friends. So I appreciated all the questions she asked and understood that she was invested in her job. She cared about the dogs and seemed to care about whether or not I was making the right decision.

I'd only known her over the phone for forty minutes, but there was something about the confidence in her voice that made me trust her. I really believed she understood what I was saying and that she had my best interest in mind.

"Look," I said, "maybe I should just get an overweight middle-aged dog, so at least we'll have something in common."

She chuckled at that—but it also seemed to strike a chord.

"You know," Casaundra said, "I might have the perfect dog for you. He's in foster care right now. Let me make a phone call and see how he's doing and I'll call you back tomorrow."

"OK, great," I said.

And with that, it was time to make dinner. I was *starving*.

I quickly read the instructions for the rice and was disappointed to see that it would take forty minutes to cook. I added two cups of rice and some water to a small pot, brought it to a boil, put a lid on it, and reduced the heat to "simmer," which I assumed was something a little less than a boil. I figured a burner setting of five would accomplish the task, and when I checked it five minutes in, the water was bubbling without boiling, so I felt pretty good about it.

While I waited for that to cook, I Googled "how to cook broccoli." The first method that popped up was blanching, which seemed way too complicated. Boil it in water, then place it in an ice bath? The second way I saw to cook broccoli was steaming, and I realized I had a steaming pan in the back of my pile of pans. It came as part of a cheap set I picked up years ago and I'd never used, not even once. I set it up, put some water in the bottom part, turned the burner on high, cut the big thick part of the broccoli stems off as suggested (which seemed like an awful waste of food), threw the broccoli into the top part of the pan with the holes in the bottom, put a lid on it, and turned my attention to the beans.

At this point I realized I had completely forgotten to look at the recipe for rice and beans on Dr. Preeti's list. I checked it out and quickly saw that I'd neglected to pick up any spices in my rush to get out of the grocery store. I also realized that the recipe called for cooking the rice and beans together in a slow cooker. *Whoops.* I hoped that cooking them separately and stirring them together would have the same result. I mean, how complicated could it be?

One of the cans of beans I picked up was labeled "baked beans." I hadn't really considered what that meant in the store, but I was glad now. I figured those must have some flavor to them. I read the ingredients and sure enough, they had plenty of "seasonings" and "natural flavors." They also had something I didn't expect: pork.

*Huh.*

These beans weren't vegetarian. That struck me as strange. Why would they sell non-vegetable vegetables? I thought a can of beans would just be beans. Seems pretty obvious. Why wouldn't it say "beans and pork" on the front of the label somewhere? I never would have known had I not read the fine print. What if this was something more important? What if I was allergic to pork, or I couldn't eat pork for religious reasons? It seemed like deceptive labeling to me.

I debated whether to go ahead and use them anyway, but decided not to. I'd already strayed far enough from Dr. Preeti's orders. So I heated up a can of plain red beans instead. The ingredients list on the can only had one ingredient: kidney beans. I hoped that didn't mean they were made from animal kidneys!

I didn't have another small or medium pot in my set, so I put them in a bowl and heated them in the microwave. Within a minute they had splattered all over the inside of the microwave, making a huge mess that I was definitely not looking forward to cleaning up. I closed the door and let them sit there so they wouldn't get cold while I waited for the rice and broccoli. I decided to eat an apple in the meantime. Then I sliced up an orange and ate that, too. I liked orange juice, but I hadn't eaten a whole orange since I was in elementary school. Oddly enough, I remembered the bitter taste of the white parts between the sections like it was yesterday, so I did my best to eat around them. It tasted great, but the whole sticky experience of sucking out the juice was tedious. I had to wash my hands afterward. *What a pain*, I thought. *Why don't they just sell these prepeeled?*

With about ten minutes left to go on the rice, I noticed the steam leaking out from under the lid looked more like smoke. I pulled the lid off and sure enough, a big puff of light-brown smoke suddenly filled my kitchen. I was shocked to find every ounce of water in that pot was gone. As I took it off the burner, the smoke detector went off. The screeching "beep, beep, beep, beep, beep!" came ripping at my eardrums as a horrible burned smell erupted from the pot.

"Damn it!" I yelled, grabbing Dr. Preeti's recipe list and using it to fan the smoke away from the detector. I quickly ran to open the door to my balcony. This was a huge building full of condos. I knew if that detector kept going off for more than a minute it would trip the building-wide system, forcing a whole building full of people to evacuate and the fire department to show up. At dinnertime.

I could picture all of my neighbors' blaming eyes fixed on me: the fat guy from apartment 313.

*Great, this is all I need.*

Thankfully my frantic fanning worked. The screeching stopped.

I turned back to the pot full of rice and found nothing but a chunky pile of mush surrounded by a burned crust. The rice at the bottom of the pan had burned so thoroughly, I couldn't scrape it off with a metal spoon. And the rice in the middle was barely cooked.

"Damn it!" I yelled, realizing I'd let the broccoli steam for that whole time. I took the steamer pan off the burner, opened it up, and saw what looked like a pile of disintegrating, wilted little trees breathing their last gasps of life. At least it was still green. It wasn't burned. I hoped it was still "good for me."

I scooped as much of the semi-cooked, non-burned rice as I could from the middle of the pot onto a plate and mixed the beans from the microwave right into it. I spooned the broccoli onto the plate, too. I tried a bite of each and it took me right back to boot camp in the army: I was eating a tray of unrecognizable slop. *This is worse than what they serve in jails,* I thought. Especially the texture.

I could not believe how badly I'd messed this up.

I doused everything with salt and pepper and made myself eat every last bite as a punishment.

If I wanted this to work, I needed to do better.

Dr. Preeti had taken an hour and a half with me in her office. She seemed like she really cared about what I was saying and what I needed to do in order to start feeling better. Casaundra had spent nearly an hour with me on the phone just trying to figure out what kind of a dog would be best suited for me and my lifestyle. And here I'd gone and rushed through this whole process of cooking my first new meal, as if I didn't care about the person I was serving it to at all.

I got up and hand-washed my dishes. I figured I'd already had twenty minutes of exercise in the grocery store, and washing dishes by hand sort of seemed like exercise, too. The burned rice left black marks on the bottom of the pot. I couldn't get them out. I scrubbed hard, but eventually just threw the pan in the garbage. It was ruined, but it was just a cheap aluminum pot. I made a mental note that I needed to buy some better cookware—and to make sure I Googled the words "how to cook" before attempting to follow any more cooking directions from the back of some package.

Over the course of the next hour, while I sat on the couch and watched TV, I forced myself to eat every last orange and apple and banana I had purchased, just to fill me up. Dr. Preeti said not to count calories, so I didn't. I didn't worry about the quantity of food I stuffed into my face. I just stuffed.

Even then it wasn't very much food. Not compared to two extra-large pizzas, anyway. For some reason I didn't feel like I had to immediately lie down and go to sleep after I ate, which is why when I finally got up to go to bed I was surprised that I didn't feel the usual tightness in my stomach— that clenching, sort-of acidic feeling I got whenever I was hungry. It was bedtime. I was *always* hungry at bedtime. If I didn't grab a snack before brushing my teeth, I went to bed dreaming about what I was going to eat for breakfast in the morning.

On this night, I felt surprisingly full.

*Huh*, I thought. *That's weird.*

# chapter 4

# First Encounters

I had a headache. My stomach hurt, too. My knees and ankles were sore from making laps around the local Petco store. My back hurt from lifting the big bag of expensive dog food into the cart and from the cart into my trunk. Still, there was something exciting about walking up to Humane Society Silicon Valley's front door knowing I would be walking out with a dog.

Casaundra had called me back just before noon, absolutely certain that she had the perfect dog for me. She gave me a list of basic stuff to buy: a dog bed, leash, water and food bowls, and so on, and told me to come in to fill out some paperwork that afternoon. The plan was to meet with her and to go through some final questions, after which, if everything went well, I would get to meet my dog.

The whole "if everything went well" part made me nervous. Casaundra took it all so seriously, there was a part of me that wondered if I was up to the task of becoming a "parent" to one of these "children."

I also wished I felt a little better. I'd woken up feeling fine, and I'd eaten plenty of oatmeal and fruit for breakfast. I didn't even put cream in my coffee. I drank it like a true road warrior: black. But something was definitely upsetting my stomach now, and with the headache on top of it, I hoped I wasn't coming down with a bug.

Humane Society Silicon Valley's facility was way more impressive than I imagined it would be. They referred to it as an Animal Community Center, and it felt more like a school campus than an animal shelter. There were volunteers playing with dogs in fenced-off playgrounds by the parking lot, and a nice concrete walkway with trees and a fountain led up to a gigantic, modern-looking building made of reddish brick, glass, and metal.

Inside, everything was clean and shining, like a newly built high school might be, and I was immediately greeted by big smiles. I let the young clerk at the front desk know I had an appointment with Casaundra, and she asked me to take a seat. One of the staff had a dog lying at her feet behind the counter while she worked at a computer. I thought, *This must be a pretty cool job for a dog lover.*

The young woman I spoke with got on the phone with Casaundra, and when she hung up she came out from behind the counter and handed me a clipboard. I sat there for quite a while filling out all of the paperwork, with background information and work history and contact numbers. It was as detailed as something you might fill out in a doctor's office.

When I turned it in, they asked if they could take a copy of my driver's license.

"Wow. You guys are thorough!" I said.

"We are," she said. "Are you excited?"

"I am. Nervous, too. I've never owned a dog before."

"Really? I've never *not* had a dog. Even when I was little. I can't even imagine life without a dog," she said.

"I just hope it likes me," I said.

"I'm sure he'll love you," she replied.

That seemed like a funny word to use: "love." Did dogs really "love"? How would you know?

"Casaundra will be out in just a minute," she added.

When she walked in, Casaundra looked nothing like I expected. Based on the sound of her voice and her professionalism over the phone, I expected someone who looked more—how should I put this?—conservative, like a banker or a schoolteacher. Instead, I found myself looking at a woman with spikey black hair, lots of tattoos, and piercings. She had a very urban look about her, as if she could hold her own in a tough neighborhood in Oakland, which reminded me that we should never judge someone on their appearance. (Or, apparently, their voice!) She smiled and shook my hand. She seemed genuinely warm and excited to see me. And when she took me back to her office, she didn't just have one dog at her feet, she had seven! Seven little dogs, all dressed in little sweaters or lying on fluffy blankets. I soon learned that all of them were at or near the end of their lives, or had some sort of illness, or had suffered some kind of abuse and were considered unadoptable. They all flocked around her the moment we walked in through the little half-door to her office, and then they came flocking around me. I felt like a little kid surrounded by a sea of puppies. They were all so sweet. I sat down on a chair and reached down to pet them, and they licked my hands and ran back and forth between me and Casaundra all excited. It felt like we'd turned their office space into a full-blown puppy party just by showing up.

This woman with the tough exterior had made it her mission to minister to the cast-off dogs of Silicon Valley—to make sure they lived comfortably and happily in their final days. She took them home with her every night and brought them into the office with her every day, so they were never alone.

"Oh, yeah," another worker said, popping her head in from the hallway to see what all the commotion was about. "She's always got six or eight of these guys. Casaundra's our resident angel, that's for sure."

We spoke for a few minutes, and I'm sure I spent a little too much time staring at the floor, or staying focused on the dogs instead of making eye contact. I was really worried that she might reject me at that point. Especially when she asked me, once again, whether I was sure I was committed to doing this. The thing is, as I petted those little dogs and saw how joyful they were, and I saw how much joy they brought to Casaundra, I felt more sure than ever. So I looked into Casaundra's eyes, and I meant it when I said, "Absolutely. Yes."

I didn't know how it would work. I didn't understand how this was really going to help me lose weight or "get healthy." But I trusted that I was following the signs I was supposed to follow. After all, the signs had now led me to an angel.

Casaundra took me into a waiting room with a door on each side. There was nothing in the room but a chair and a bench. The single window was frosted, so it let light in but you couldn't see anything through it. The gray concrete floor had a drain in the center.

"Now, you know how to greet a dog you've never met, right?" she said.

"No, I guess not."

"Just put your hand out like this, with your wrist down, and your fingers in more of a fist. You don't want them sticking out where they could get bit," she said.

*Is this dog going to bite me?* I wondered.

I mirrored her motions. "Also, put your head down a little, look down at the ground, so the dog doesn't think you're trying to dominate him. Don't look him in the eyes at first." I knew that wouldn't be a problem for me. "Be a little submissive so he knows he's safe. You might want to sit. Let him sniff your hand, and then the best thing is to really just let the dog come to you. You don't want to try to pet him right away. Just give him a second. He's a real sweet dog once he knows you."

*Once he knows me?* I thought. *That doesn't sound like the happy eight-pound golden retriever I came for.*

"All right. You ready to meet the perfect dog for you?"

"Ready as I'll ever be," I said.

Casaundra stepped out of the room, and I took a deep breath. My heart was pounding.

I sat in that little isolation chamber with nothing but anticipation, and then I heard footsteps approaching. Dog nails on concrete. The handle on the door turned. The door cracked open. A black nose tried to push its way in first, and then Casaundra opened the door all the way. There he was:

a large black-and-white dog with a big round body, shuffling into the room with his head hung low. He looked up at me and then dropped his head with a clear look of disappointment. Like, "*Really? This* loser? *Did you walk me into the wrong room?*"

I suppose I looked at him the same way.

All I could think was, *This is not the dog I imagined at all.*

"Eric, meet Raider. Raider, this is Eric," Casaundra said.

"Raider?" I asked.

"Like the Oakland Raiders. His owners were fans. And he's black and white, so…"

The Raiders were my least favorite sports team on the planet. I had friends who referred to themselves as "Raider haters."

I put my hand out just as she instructed and looked down at the floor. I felt his wet nose touch my knuckles, and only then did I look him in the eyes again. I swear he was still eyeing me with disappointment—probably because I was looking at him the same way. This dog just looked depressed. I don't think I'd ever seen a depressed dog before, but that's definitely what he looked like to me. And he was not a small dog. In addition to being plump, he came up to my knees. He had to be a good seventy-five pounds. His fur was all scruffy and matted in spots, and he seemed like a dog that was the very opposite of joyful.

"What kind of a dog is he?"

"He's a border collie and Australian shepherd mix, to the best of our knowledge," Casaundra said.

"Oh, wow. Aren't those, like, super-energetic breeds? Don't they require all kinds of exercise?"

"Normally, yes. They're great agility dogs. But as you can see, he's a middle-aged, overweight dog, just like you asked for, and that means he's in need of a new routine, just like the one you told me you needed. I wouldn't want you to leave here with a dog that's in great shape who needs to go running every day, because it wouldn't be a match, you know? Raider's kinda slow moving. He's out of shape. His joints are swollen. He needs to start walking again, which is very in line with what your doctor wants for you, correct?"

"Yeah, I guess," I said. "How old is he?"

"He is seven."

Casaundra let him off leash while we spoke, and Raider was just sort of sniffing around the perimeter of the room. I wondered how many other dogs had come through there, and I wondered how many other humans, like me, were skeptical of the results of this whole dog-human match-making process.

I didn't want to let Casaundra down. I knew that she'd really put some thought and effort into this, and it was meaningful to her. I thought, *This is what she does for a living, and she really feels strongly about this. I'm sure she isn't trying to pawn this dog off on me because I'm an easy mark. And perhaps this is another "sign."*

I tried to give her the benefit of the doubt.

"Why did someone give this dog up?" I asked.

Casaundra flipped through a few pages of notes on a clipboard. "There was a divorce. He was not being cared for the way that he needed. He spent a lot of time in a backyard by himself after his primary caregiver went off to college. And the family just felt like maybe there was a better home for him somewhere else," Casaundra said.

After making his way around the perimeter, Raider came over and sniffed my shoes. He looked up, and I reached out to pet him behind the ears. He sort of flopped his head down and leaned into it, so I scratched a little harder. He seemed to like that. When I stopped for a moment, he lay down on the floor near my feet. I leaned over and petted him some more.

"Aw, look at that. He likes you already," Casaundra said. "So, a few things to know about Raider. His behavior assessment says no children, due to a history of being nervous and frightened of children and older teens. And so that's one reason I thought your home might be good for him, because you live alone. When he first got here, he was really stressed. He avoided people. He wasn't interested in treats. He was giving us the whale eye. That means he was, you know, giving us some warnings, like, 'Don't come near me.' It was obvious he couldn't handle this environment, with all of these other dogs around."

"Wow," I said. I was impressed by just how much thought they put into how the dog felt, being thrust into that situation.

"It says here that he was attacked by a German shepherd as a puppy, and was especially aggressive toward that breed because of that, but he was also leash-reactive in general, meaning he barked at other dogs and other people whenever he was on leash. He just needed to get to a better environment, and so I decided to place him in foster care. We do matchmaking for that, too, and Melissa, who I placed him with, is a professional in terms of handling animals. She doesn't foster many dogs, but she has a real love for these herding breeds, and she doesn't have kids, so it was a good fit."

"And how did he do with her?"

"So, you know, once I got him in Melissa's home, his stress level went way down. I have notes in here that show he's doing well. He's crate trained and potty trained. When he's unleashed in a controlled area, he loves going outside. He doesn't jump on people, not mouthy, knows basic commands. He does bark at people, and is *very* focused on stray cats, this says. Oh, they took him out to a cabin. It says he's doing well with other dogs, although, in that house he had an issue with one of them. He's a good hiker, loved the snow. So, you know, he's doing well, and that's after being in foster for only about ten days."

"Yeah?"

"Yeah. Being in a quiet home like yours, starting slowly, I think he'll do really well. I think you'll both do really well. I have a good feeling about this," she said to me. "Just be patient and give it some time. You have to understand that his whole life has been uprooted. He had a family situation that changed, which caused him stress, but it was still his family that left him here. And that family had adopted him from a shelter when he was younger, too. So he's gone through two families now, two adoptions, plus the trauma of coming here, and then adjusting to a foster home—it's going to take him some time to adjust."

"The poor guy," I said. It suddenly hit me how tough this dog's life had been. Imagine being a part of a family and having that family abandon you, only to have another family give up on you, too. I don't know why it hit me the way it did. I'd never really had any empathy for the plight of animals. I wasn't a Greenpeace or PETA kind of guy, or someone who even felt sad about those animal adoption commercials on TV. Not that I didn't care about animals, I just never spent a whole lot of time thinking about them.

I looked down at Raider and suddenly the sadness in his eyes didn't look like a reflection on me. It looked more like weariness. Heartache. Maybe loneliness. A feeling like he was just done and ready to give up and die.

Like me.

I started to tear up. I could hardly believe it.

Raider rolled on his side and started panting a little bit as I began petting him. It wasn't hot in that room, so it seemed concerning. "Is he OK?" I asked.

"Yeah, I think he's just a little stressed. Dogs smell the stress of other dogs in this room. This is also a room where families come to surrender their dogs, so there's a lot of emotion in here."

I looked at him, petting him in silence for a bit.

"Can I ask you something?" I said.

"Of course."

"Can I change his name?"

"Why?" Casaundra asked.

"Look, I'm from the South Bay. I live in Forty-Niners country. I'm a Forty-Niners fan. We hate the Raiders. I just—"

Casaundra laughed. "I get it!" she said. "Yes, you can change his name. It might take him a while to respond, but why not? Fresh start."

"Yeah?"

"Absolutely. He'll adjust. He'll adjust…"

"Well," I said. "Then I guess that's that."

"All right!" Casaundra said. "I really feel good about you two. I really think you'll start off on the right foot together. Just have patience. Take those walks. Don't go too far, though. Don't try to, like, show him around and take him all sorts of places with you right away. Don't go any farther than he needs to go to go to the bathroom for the first couple of weeks. Start slow, and you'll both be OK."

"Starting slow sounds good to me. Yeah. Thank you, Casaundra."

"You're welcome, Eric. Thank *you*. Raider thanks you. Oh, and because of his behavioral stuff, we would like you to take some classes with him. It'll help you both to bond and ultimately make the transition easier for both of you. They're not too expensive, and well worth it," she said.

"I, um…OK. Whatever you say," I answered.

I put Raider on his new leash, walked him out front to complete some final paperwork, shook Casaundra's hand, and suddenly I found myself on the concrete walk, passing the fountain, headed toward my car. With a *dog*.

Raider seemed a little different the moment we got outside. He stepped out in front of me, pulling forward on the leash and moving back and forth across the walkway as if he were on patrol. He pulled hard and barked at a dog in one of the playgrounds, and it took a considerable amount of strength to hold him back and urge him to keep moving.

"Come on there, Raider. That dog can't get to you. Come on!" I said. "Raider!"

He finally moved along. "Boy, we have got to change that name. What's a good name for you, huh?"

I realized I was talking to a dog. That was weird. Why was I doing that? Did I expect him to answer?

I unlocked the car and opened the back door, expecting Raider to jump right in. But he didn't. He just stood there.

"Go on, boy. This is your new car. Hop in!"

I pulled on his leash, I even gave him a little nudge with my knee, but he looked up at me as if he'd never jumped into a car in his life. As if he had no idea what to do.

"Come on, boy, you can do it."

I finally bent down, wrapped my arms around his chest just behind his front legs, and physically lifted him up. It was awkward, and it took all of my strength, with his legs all dangling down kicking and squirming, until I finally got him onto the seat. I worried the whole time that he might try to bite me or something for manhandling him like that, but he didn't. Once he was in the car he lay down, flat, as if he didn't want to look out the window; as if he didn't care to see where he might wind up next.

I closed the door and leaned against the car. I had to catch my breath after all of the bending and lifting. I closed my eyes and felt the sun on my face and thought, *God, I sure hope this isn't a mistake.*

Even as I backed out of my space and pulled onto the street, Raider stayed down in the backseat. I'd known people with dogs that hopped all over their cars and tried to crawl into their laps while they drove, and I was very glad this dog wasn't like that. I worried about him, though. I raised my head and adjusted my rearview mirror so I could see him. He seemed to look back at me with a side-eyed glance as his head lay on his front paws.

"So, boy, what should we call you?" I asked him.

For some reason, something about the cute position he was lying in made me flash back to my childhood. Growing up, my favorite TV show was *The Little Rascals*. The gang of kids in that show had a dog named Peety. That Peety was some sort of bull dog with a big black circle around his eye, and he looked absolutely nothing like this dog in my back-seat. But they were both black and white, and I remembered way back then thinking it would be cool to have a dog like that.

Now here I was, driving home with the first dog I'd ever owned, and he was a black-and-white dog, too. It seemed like fate.

"How about Peety?" I said. "Can I call you Peety?"

I'm not sure if it was a coincidence, if he heard something or smelled something that caught his attention, or if he somehow recognized the positive childhood memories that resonated in that name when I spoke it out loud, but the moment I said "Peety," that dog raised his head and looked right at me.

I took it as another sign.

"Well that's it then," I said. "Peety, let's go home."

When we reached my building, Peety managed to waddle out of the car on his own just fine. But when the elevator door opened, he stood at the end of his leash again, staring, as if he didn't know what to do. I don't think he had ever seen an elevator before. I managed to pull him in by his collar, and I watched his head as he looked around nervously, sensing the motion of that tiny box of a room. Then the doors opened and we were in a completely different environment with nice lighting and carpeted floors. Peety looked really confused. We had entered a box in one place, and we were now exiting that box in an entirely different place. The look on his face was, "What is up with that?"

I walked him to the door of my condo and once inside, I finally let him off his leash. He plodded down the hallway, past the kitchen, all the way over by the door to the balcony on the far side of the room. He lay down and let out a big sigh as I hung his leash on my key rack.

I'd managed to carry a bag full of toys and treats up with us, but Peety's big bag of dog food and his dog bed were still in the car. I decided I was too tired to go get them. Peety looked like he didn't want to move, either, so I left him alone. I collapsed on the couch after my long day out, and I let out a big sigh myself.

Then I took a deep breath in, and my senses were suddenly overwhelmed with the most delicious scent wafting from the kitchen: the scent of a meal I had completely forgotten I'd started to prepare that morning.

Right after my oatmeal-and-coffee breakfast, I had forced myself to go out shopping again. I went to a nice kitchen store and bought myself a Crock-Pot. I bought a new set of tri-ply stainless-steel pots and pans, with thick bottoms that the salesperson insisted would help eliminate burning and distribute the heat from my stove burners more evenly. I took the salesperson's recommendation for steaming vegetables and bought a set of Asian-style steaming baskets as well. I told her about my broccoli mush, and she said, "I only steam broccoli for a couple of minutes. I like my vegetables al dente." That sounded very fancy, and I liked the sound of it. I bought some new utensils, and a bunch of little glass bowls and mixing bowls and more. Then I went back to the grocery store and bought more fruits and vegetables, and some more beans—in a bag this time, not a can. I looked at Dr. Preeti's ingredient list more closely and bought a whole rack's worth of spices. I vowed to follow her rice-and-beans recipe to a T, and I came home, measured everything out into my new little bowls—just the way you'd see a celebrity chef do on a morning TV show—and then I dumped the rice, beans, and perfectly measured spices into the Crock-Pot. I put the lid on and set it to high. It didn't make much sense to me how those raw ingredients and spices would mix and mingle into something edible by dinnertime, but I decided to just keep going with this on faith.

Lying on that couch, still a couple of hours until it was supposed to be ready, I found myself salivating. It smelled like something from an exotic Indian or Middle-Eastern restaurant. I couldn't believe I'd created something that smelled so fragrant and delicious in my own kitchen. The scent of it made my whole apartment feel fresh and new to me, just as that strange sunlight had after my little trip into the light. It filled up my senses.

I didn't really move for the next couple of hours. Neither did Peety, except every few minutes when he would scratch himself. He scratched so hard that he kept waking me up from my nap. It drove me nuts. As the afternoon sun came streaming through the windows, I noticed that his scratching sent a huge cloud of dust and dog hair into the air every time. I knew that HSSV wouldn't have let me leave with a dirty dog, which meant his dust cloud must have been made up entirely of his own dry skin.

"Eew," I said to him. "We're gonna have to do something about that."

Peety gazed at me with that weary look again.

I decided to sit up and try to play with him. I opened the Petco bag and pulled out a ball.

"You want to play? You want a ball?"

I rolled it across the floor and he followed it with his eyes, watching as it bounced off the wall and rolled under the coffee table. He didn't move an inch.

"Don't like balls, huh?"

Peety put his head back down on his front paws. I reached into the bag again and pulled out a rubber squeaky hot dog. I pressed it over and over, filling the room with squeaky sounds, and then I tossed it his way. It bounced off of his back leg and fell to the floor.

"What about a rope? You want to play tug-of-war?"

I dangled a rope toy from my fingers and shook it around, and he stared at me like I was the world's most boring clown. I tossed it across the floor to him, and once again, he didn't move.

"Well, how about a treat then," I said. Peety perked his ears up for that. I pulled a couple of dog treats from a box, stood up with a groan, and walked across the room. I placed them in the palm of my hand, got down on one knee— which was no easy feat—and placed them under his snout.

He sniffed them. Cautiously. Then he pushed his nose down into the palm of my hand and ate them.

"Good boy," I said, scratching him behind the ears. He stared at me and wagged his tail. "Does that mean you're hungry? 'Cause I know I sure am."

I pressed my left hand against the wall and lifted myself up, which forced me to stop and catch my breath again.

"Tell you what. Why don't we get our first walk over with, OK? We'll go down, you can go to the bathroom, we'll grab your food and new bed out of the car, and then we'll come up here and eat. That sound good?"

I grabbed a container of poop pickup bags from the Petco treasure stash, and no sooner had I picked up Peety's leash than Peety was up and walking right to me. I hooked the leash to his collar, opened the door, and he stepped out into the hallway ahead of me.

"Well, OK then," I said. "I guess I'll let you lead."

## chapter 5

# Cleanup Time

As soon as we cleared the elevator and stepped onto the concrete steps near the parking garage, Peety lifted his leg and peed all over the wall.

"No, boy! No!" I said, but the damage was done. It was like someone opened a fire hydrant on a hot day. I could not believe how thoroughly he soaked that wall in a matter of seconds. I was very glad there were no other residents around to witness his transgression. We lived in a pet-friendly building, but no building is *that* pet-friendly.

Peety then turned and spotted another dog being walked by a man way down at the end of the block.

"Woof! Woof, woof!" he barked, loudly, while aggressively tugging on the leash.

"No, Peety, no!" I yelled, pulling him back and trying to force him to walk in the opposite direction. He led me to the nearest tree and stopped and peed a little, and to the next tree, where he stopped and peed a little again. I took it as a good sign. He was marking his territory. Maybe he needed to do that in order to treat this as his new home.

Peety definitely took the lead. He did his side-to-side sweep again, out in front of me as he walked, sort of sweeping the sidewalk on the lookout for enemies. Lucky for me, Peety didn't walk very fast. At that point, after an already long day, I felt like I was barely lumbering along. You could practically hear my footsteps on the sidewalk as I swung each leg forward—"Thump, thump, thump," like the giant from *Jack and the Beanstalk*.

We passed a few other people on the sidewalk as we both hobbled halfway up the block. I didn't look at any of them or say anything to them. I was used to being invisible. My size automatically made me unapproachable almost everywhere I went. But Peety looked at everyone. He seemed to size them up quickly, and either ignore them or growl. It was kind of scary. I wondered if Peety could see something in people that I couldn't. I know Casaundra told me he was "leash-reactive," but I didn't quite know what it meant, until that moment. I wrapped the leash three times around my right wrist and held it tight with two hands whenever another person came anywhere near us. The last thing I needed was to have this dog bite someone and get me sued.

No one tried to pet him. No one stopped to say, "Oh, what a cute dog."

Frankly, I was glad we didn't encounter any children. I'm not sure what would have happened if some naive kid came running up and tried to hug him or something. If he was vicious, I'm sure Casaundra would have told me. But the way he walked, given how overweight he was, I'm sure his joints were in pain, just like mine were. Maybe all of him was in pain. An animal in pain that feels threatened might bite. That seemed logical to me.

Peety finally did his business in a patch of grass adjacent to our building. I picked it up in one of the little bags, which were conveniently held in a container that clipped right to the leash. (I imagined whoever invented that little bag holder was probably now a millionaire.) It was the first time I'd ever picked up a poop in my hand, and it was just about as gross as I'd anticipated. The warmth of it radiated through that thin layer of plastic, and even though I tried to be thorough, some bits of his mess got left behind on the blades of grass. I felt bad about that, but at least we lived in California, I figured, where the sprinkler system would wash it all away after dark.

Peety walked right into the elevator when we went back inside. He turned in the right direction when we came out of the elevator and led me right to the door of my condo. He certainly seemed to be a quick learner.

I, on the other hand, was a little slow sometimes.

"Oh, shoot. I forgot your food," I said. I hated when I did things like that. There were times when I felt like my mind was in a fog. I never spoke to anyone about it, but I worried that maybe I was experiencing some serious signs of early aging. And that frightened me.

I decided to let him in and go back down to the car without him. He beelined it straight for his spot on the far side of the apartment, where he'd already spent most of his afternoon.

"I'll be right back," I said, and off I went, lumbering all

the way back to the elevator and out to my car in order to heft a giant bag of dog food and a big fluffy bed all the way back to where I already was.

As I returned, two of my neighbor's kids went running down the hall, and I heard Peety barking like crazy from behind my door. It sounded like he was attacking the door, trying to get through. I couldn't believe how loud he was, like a whole pack of wolves stuffed into one body. *At least I won't have to worry about anyone robbing my apartment*, I thought.

I opened the door and the delicious scent of the rice and beans blasted me. I figured it must be fully cooked by now, and I couldn't wait to dive in. I washed my hands, poured Peety some dog food, and watched as he came sauntering into the kitchen. He ate it all in a matter of seconds and then stared up at me, like, "Dude. Fill 'er up!"

It seemed like a lot of food to me, and sure enough, I read the bag and realized I'd given him more than the recommended amount for a dog his size. But I knew he needed to lose weight, so I didn't refill his bowl.

"Sorry, boy. Have some water. You'll have to wait until breakfast," I said.

I finally took the lid off the Crock-Pot and I could not believe how amazingly rich and tantalizing that rice-and-beans concoction looked. OK, maybe I was just starving. I hadn't eaten since breakfast. And I still thought of it as a side dish, not a main course, but all of the spices that were just sort of scattered on the top had magically blended down into the rice in that pot, and the aromas that filled my apartment were matched by this wonderful reddish-brown color, and a weighty, sticky texture that clung to my wooden spoon as I dished it onto my plate.

I put a forkful of it right up to my nose and savored the scent of it up close, one last time, before I finally put it in my mouth. The taste was so amazing that I actually closed my eyes and chewed it in slow-motion ecstasy.

"Wow, that's good!" I exclaimed.

Peety was now sitting there staring up at me.

"Yeah. OK. You've gotta try this," I said to him, and I put a forkful in his bowl. He inhaled it.

"Isn't that amazing?"

I could not believe that I was calling a dish made of nothing but rice and beans "amazing." Let alone a dish that I'd made in my own kitchen. But it was!

My Crock-Pot was the largest model available, and I'd made enough for probably three or four big meals—but I went ahead and dished out a whole second serving, cleaning out more than half the pot in one sitting and swallowing every bit of it with just as much joy as I'd experienced on the very first bite.

"Man, that was good," I said. "What do you think, Peety? You think we can do this?"

Peety didn't answer of course. Once my plate was empty and he realized he wasn't getting any more food, he sauntered off toward his spot.

"Wait, wait. Hold on, boy," I said. I popped up and grabbed his new bed, which I'd left by the door, and laid it out right there in the spot he seemed to like best. He stepped right into it, circled himself around a couple of times, and plopped down with yet another great big sigh.

I went in and did the dishes by hand again, figuring I probably hadn't hit my exercise quota for the day. But as I washed the dishes, I looked at the clock and did some math. I'd walked around two different stores that morning, for a solid forty minutes in the kitchen store, and ten or fifteen minutes in the grocery store. Oh! And then the trip to Petco. That was another half hour on my feet. I'd also walked to and from the HSSV parking lot. I'd then walked Peety for fifteen minutes or so outside, and then walked back and forth to my car to get his stuff. So I'd done *way* more than two twenty-minute stints of exercise already, and now I was standing up scrubbing the dishes.

"Forget that!" I said. I threw them all into the dishwasher instead.

I wasn't even a full day into this thing, and having Peety around had kept me moving far more than I ever would have on a normal day.

I wound up eating an apple while I watched TV that night. Just one apple. I drank a couple of big glasses of water because I was a lot more thirsty than normal. I think that was due to one of the spices in the rice and beans. I'm not sure. And when I went to bed, I noticed once again that I wasn't hungry.

*Huh*, I thought.

The next morning I woke up with a craving—for rice and beans. I had never eaten any food remotely like that before noon, and yet on that morning, that's what I wanted.

I threw some clothes on and took Peety out first, fearing he might really have to go bad after being inside the whole night. As we exited the elevator I tried to hurry him along toward the grass—but once again, the moment we stepped onto the concrete steps, he unleashed like a fire hose.

"Peety!" I yelled, a little bit exaggerated for the sake of one of my neighbors who was on his way into the building. "I'm sorry," I said, not making eye contact. "New dog."

"Oh, yeah?" the man said. "He doesn't look new."

The guy couldn't have been much over thirty. I'd seen him around before but never spoken to him.

"Yeah, well, I got him at a shelter just yesterday. I haven't had a chance to train him yet," I said.

"Oh, wow. That's a nice thing, to adopt an older dog like that. Very cool, man. Good luck with him."

I looked up, and the guy was smiling.

"Thanks," I said.

We spoke more words than I'd exchanged with any neighbor in that building since I'd moved in. It was a nice building in what used to be a pretty bad neighborhood in East San Jose. It was a mostly Hispanic area, in the same zip code where Cesar Chavez grew up. I was definitely a minority here, and the building itself stood out from the older, smaller buildings all around it. The developers were sort of pioneers, and because of that, it was one of the only nice new condos I could afford in the whole overpriced region.

I had never walked out onto the sidewalk before. I always went straight from the elevator to my car and vice versa. I purposefully avoided talking to anyone, less out of any sort of fear than because I had learned to avoid people in general. So the whole exchange felt strange to me. And the fact that the man smiled instead of getting mad about a dog peeing all over our nice building was just astounding to me.

I walked Peety all the way to the end of the block and back that morning. We walked slowly, as he sniffed every tree and rock along the way. We put in our full twenty minutes before we headed back upstairs. The funny thing was, I was craving those rice and beans so much I didn't even stop to collapse on the couch after all that walking. I poured Peety his food and he gobbled it up, and I threw a big helping of my concoction in the microwave.

Even reheated, the rice and beans were *that good*. I ate them all. I felt full.

I didn't want to forget about the half-a-plate-of-fruits-and-vegetables part of the equation, so I also ate an orange and a banana, then promised myself I'd steam some broccoli that night—al dente—in my new bamboo steamers. I also vowed to read up on "how to steam broccoli" again on the Internet, just to be sure I didn't mess it up.

Over the course of working the phones and e-mailing clients that day, I read some food blogs and caught a little nutrition tip that sounded simple enough to follow: "Eat the rainbow." The idea was to eat foods of every color over the course of your day. I had never thought about the colors of foods, but when I thought about my regular diet, most of it was kind of beige and brown. Hamburgers, chicken, pasta. Eggs at least had some yellow, and spaghetti sauce was red, but there just wasn't a whole lot of color in general. Already that morning I'd consumed orange, red, and dark-red/purplish colors in the rice dish, and I planned on covering green that night. About the only color missing was blue. *I ought to pick up some blueberries today*, I thought, and I made a mental note to stop by the grocery store again.

I also made a mental note to ask Dr. Preeti about this rainbow idea, and somehow, I was sure she would approve.

I tried to get Peety to play with a ball or a toy again. He just wasn't interested. After two days and nights together, he didn't seem much interested in anything except peeing on the concrete, eating, and sleeping in his spot. But then on the third night, something changed. No sooner had I turned out the light than I heard Peety's footsteps waddling across the living room floor. He walked into my bedroom, jumped on the bed, made a couple of circles, and then curled up right next to me.

"Well, hey, boy," I said. He let out a sigh as I shook the whole bed while turning myself over to put my arm around him. I petted him in long strokes, from the top of his head all the way down his back. I could feel the warmth of his body through the covers, and you know what? It felt good.

"You getting used to me now?" I asked.

Peety made a sort of sighing moan that I took as a "yes," and I laughed a little.

"Well, good," I said.

I could feel him drift off to sleep as I continued to pet him, and shortly thereafter I fell asleep, too, with my big arm wrapped right over him.

He would sleep in my bed every night from that day forward.

There was just one problem with that: Peety's shedding was out of control. He woke me up multiple times every night with his scratching. The pre-dog worries I had about an apartment and business clothes covered in dog hair came true—only tenfold. I had never encountered a dog that shed this much in my life. My entire bed was *covered* in Peety fur. It scattered across the floor like tumbleweeds on a windy day whenever I took a step. It clung to my bare toes and the soles of my feet when I got out of the shower.

I had to do something. Not only was it driving me nuts, but I could tell Peety wasn't comfortable in his own skin. I knew what that was like. Not just because of my weight, but because I'd long suffered from plaque psoriasis—a red, scaly, miserable skin condition that would flare up and linger at times, in all different parts of my body. It caused itching and sometimes pain that wouldn't go away. I'd sought treatment for years, and nothing worked. So watching Peety scratch himself, seeing his flaky skin and his hair flying around, pained me.

I decided to take action.

The first thing I decided to do was to hire a cleaning person.

Knowing that somebody else was going to step foot into my apartment made me spring into action. I spent hours picking up and organizing the place just so I wouldn't be embarrassed. It seemed ridiculous that I was cleaning to impress my new cleaning lady, but I had to do it. I bought a box full of large industrial-grade garbage bags, the solid black kind that no one could see through. I filled them up with all of the used socks and underwear that were piled in the spare bedroom. It took me multiple trips to heft all of those bags down to the Dumpster. I was a sweaty mess and collapsed on the couch when it was all over. But it was done. Those mountains were gone.

Celia, who preferred to be called Sally, showed up for her first visit later that week and spent eight hours turning my apartment into a crystal palace. I had never lived anyplace so clean. After vacuuming up all the hair, inch by inch, she removed stains that I didn't even know were there: the discoloration on the floor of the tub, greasy finger stains on light switches. She even cleaned the baseboards and made the stainless steel in the kitchen shine. Peety really liked her, too. He seemed to like having a woman in the place. He followed her from room to room as she worked. I heard her squeal once, and I called from the kitchen to ask if something was wrong.

"No, no," Sally said. She was laughing. "I was just down on the floor and Peety came up and licked my foot!"

Right after I hired Sally, the second thing I did was to take Peety on a visit back to HSSV. They had a pet supply shop there at the facility, and I figured if I was going to spend money on some kind of remedies, and maybe some new toys while I was at it, I'd prefer to give my money to them.

Casaundra happened to be up at the front desk as Peety and I walked in—and she could not hide the look of dread on her face.

"Hi, Eric! Hi, Raider!" she said in feigned excitement. "What brings you two back?"

I realized why she was concerned: she was worried I'd given up. She was terrified that I was bringing Peety back to surrender and drop him off.

"Hi! No, no, his name's Peety now. We're just here to do some shopping," I said.

The smile that came over Casaundra's face was glorious.

"Oh, good! Good. How's everything going?"

She and the other folks behind the counter all came around to greet Peety, and petted him, and he seemed to love all of the attention.

"We're pretty good. Except his skin condition is just awful. He's scratching all the time. Shedding like you can't believe. I'm not sure what to do," I said.

"I'll go ask one of our vets what they recommend. It's so good to see you, Peety," she said. And off she went. Peety and I went into the store and I immediately spotted another dog in there with its owner. I triple-wrapped the leash around my wrist and prepared for Peety to freak out. But he didn't. He didn't react at all. When that dog came closer, they both sniffed each other out and moved on. It was bizarre.

I took Peety to look at some toys, hoping something would strike his fancy. He ignored just about everything until he saw this one toy called a Kong. It was a red rubbery ball-like thing that was hollow in the middle and had a thick red rope running through it. He put his nose right up to it on the rack and nudged it.

"You like that?"

That one toy was almost twenty dollars. But it was the first interest he'd shown in any kind of toy, so I thought he should have it.

"You have expensive tastes, huh? I used to be like that," I said.

"So, Eric," Casaundra said as she walked in behind me. "They recommend you add some oil to his food. We have a product right here," she said, grabbing a little bottle of food additive. "The only problem they see with that is that he's already overweight. This adds a lot of calories and fat. But you might try it, and hopefully the condition will improve a little and you can wean him off it as he loses weight with exercise. You're walking, right?"

"We are. Every day. Still just down the block and back, like you recommended. But we may branch out a little farther next week."

"Good! I'm so glad it's going well."

"It really is. He sort of kept his distance the first couple of days, but then on the third night he jumped up into my bed and has slept there right next to me ever since."

"See, I told you! Just give it time. He's a good boy, aren't you, Peety?"

Peety looked up at her and started panting a little, with his tongue out, all pink and cute. She petted him on the head.

"I've got to go. We've got a surrender coming in. Feel free to call me with any questions or anything," she said.

"I will. Thank you again," I said.

We paid for our things, and no sooner did we step outside onto the concrete than we saw another couple walking in with a pit bull. Peety went nuts! I had let my guard down in the store and unwound the leash from my wrist, and I almost lost him.

"Whoa, boy. No!" I shouted. "Sit!" I pulled the leash as he yanked so hard he lifted his front legs right off the ground. The couple with the pit bull hurried their way inside, and Peety calmed down as soon as they were out of sight.

"Peety, sit!" I said. And he sat. "Peety, you cannot do that. Why were you so calm with the dog in the store and so angry at this other one, huh? No, boy. Just...no."

I added some of the oil to his food that night, but I was scared at the idea that it might cause him to put on even more weight. He was already seventy-five pounds. He should have been *fifty*.

As for my weight? I would soon learn that the shift to plant-based food had done me surprisingly well.

# chapter 6

# Going Plant-Based

At my second office visit with Dr. Preeti, I checked in five pounds lighter than I'd weighed the week before.

"I'm actually surprised it's not more," I said, "because I *feel* different. I feel lighter."

"Yes, well, it's not all about the numbers," Dr. Preeti said. "Have you eliminated meats and animal products entirely?"

"Almost," I said. "I broke down a couple of nights and ate the tuna, from the cans you gave me as an allowance. I ate two cans each night, so I only have two left. But I didn't mix them up with mayonnaise or anything. I just added some salt and pepper and put them on top of a salad. Did you know they make salad mixes that are already pre-washed and ready to eat? With all sorts of greens?"

"Yes. They're expensive. I prefer to buy whole greens and then make up a salad myself, but that's really, really good. What else have you been eating?"

"Well, no pizza. Only a couple of drive-throughs when I was out visiting clients. I got some french fries. I figured they're a vegetable, and you said don't worry about counting calories, so I figured it was OK," I said.

"No burgers or chicken?"

"No! None. I think I did good!"

"That's fantastic."

"And I followed your rice-and-beans recipe, for the slow cooker, and it was delicious. I ate it pretty much every night. Even for breakfast a couple of times."

"Wow! Eric, that's so great. A lot of clients don't follow the advice I give them, and then wonder why it's not working, you know? I'm just so glad you tried to follow your plan and do your best. What else? What were your other breakfasts?"

"I did eat some toast, but with jelly, no butter. And oatmeal, and coffee."

"Ah," she said.

"How did you feel on the days you ate bread?"

"What do you mean?"

"How did you feel after eating bread as compared to days with no bread?"

"Hmmm. Well... I haven't really thought about how I felt after a particular meal. In general, I usually feel tired after I eat. What do you mean?"

"Have you had any problems as you've switched to this diet? Headaches, stomach, bowels—"

"Yes," I said. "Some killer headaches. Definitely some stomach and bowel issues. I figure that's because I'm getting so much fiber in these fruit and vegetables."

"Well, fiber will make you more regular, but will not typically cause stomach and bowel discomfort. You've been reading up on this, I take it?"

"I have. Tons of research. Reading up on cooking techniques. Trying to understand."

"Well, here's why I ask. Your blood work came back and, in addition to a number of other issues, it does show markers for gluten sensitivity."

"Gluten sensitivity?"

"Yes, which is why I'm wondering how you felt after eating toast at breakfast, and fast-food french fries."

"Gluten's in wheat, right? The stuff that binds bread, and pastas, and—"

"Yes."

"I read about that. It seems like there's a lot of hype around it."

"Yes, there is a lot of controversy in the medical community about gluten and how it may affect people differently."

I asked if I could look at the calendar on her wall, and I thought back to the breakfast I had after my first, disastrous rice-and-beans attempt: six slices of toast—and I wound up with a screaming headache that day.

"Yeah. You might be onto something," I said.

"So, in addition to meats and animal products, for this next week I'd like you to try to avoid gluten. I think I had recommended that you avoid bread, anyway. It was on the list of foods I asked you to avoid, wasn't it?"

"It was. But since it wasn't a meat product, I wasn't sure why. So I just went ahead and ate it."

"Bread is a calorie-dense, processed food. It's not a whole, plant-based food, and most commercially available breads include many different ingredients. Chances are that store-bought bread contains eggs, plus added sugar and butter or margarine or oil."

"Oh. I didn't even consider that," I said.

"It can be tricky. And gluten, whether or not it's a problem for you, is used in many different foods, where you would least expect it. Especially prepackaged and processed foods. It shows up in some brands of corn tortillas, and even french fries," she said.

"French fries are potatoes," I countered.

"Not always. French fries served by many restaurants, and especially fast-food restaurants, are often made from a paste, like a dough that is made from ground-up potatoes and gluten and other binders and flavorings, which is shaped to look like a french fry. In fact, some fast-food fries aren't even vegetarian," she said.

"What?"

"Some are flavored with beef broth."

"You're kidding. What if someone's allergic to this stuff? How are they supposed to know?"

"You need to ask if you aren't certain. As another example, many restaurants prepare rice using chicken broth. The only way to know is to ask for an ingredient list or ask your server to make sure that all food you order is what you think it is and does not include any unwanted ingredients."

"Wow," I said. "Wow. OK. So no more bread. And I'll try to watch for gluten, too, and see if it makes a difference."

"Don't stress out over it. Just try. See how it goes. If you feel better, then continue. And go ahead and have those last cans of tuna if you want and see if you can be one hundred percent plant-based after that as well. I think it will make a real difference."

"It already has. I mean, I really do feel so much lighter. It's hard to explain. Especially since I haven't lost much weight," I said.

"We'll talk more as you get used to it, and about some other things, too. Cutting back on sugars. Oils. All of these things that may be causing your body stress."

"Oils, huh?" I thought of Peety. "I don't eat a lot of sugar."

"You might be surprised. There's sugar in so many things that we aren't aware of, too."

"Like gluten and beef broth?"

"Yes."

"That's deceptive labeling, isn't it? I mean, shouldn't manufacturers and restaurants clearly label what's in their food? Shouldn't we be told what we're putting in our bodies?"

"If only they would, it would be much easier. Yes."

"To be frank, I'm a little worried that I'm eliminating too many foods now, though. What will be left for me to eat? I've enjoyed the rice and beans, but I'm already kind of sick of them. I need more variety."

"Have you tried any of the other recipes I gave you?"

"No, not really. I don't know what some of this stuff is. Quin-oh? Quin—"

"Quinoa," she said. I had no idea it was pronounced "keen-wa" until that very moment.

"Right. And tofu. I had tofu once, years ago, and it was just slimy and awful. I can't possibly eat that. And so many of these things—"

"Well, if you can, just try. There are lots of vegan cook-books out there. And try not to think about what you're giving up, but instead think about what you're gaining, including your health. There are more than twenty thousand edible plants on earth. The list of things you *can* eat is far longer than the short list of things you can't."

"Twenty thousand? That's crazy. I can count the list of vegetables I've eaten in my entire life on two hands. I mean, I had forgotten I liked corn. I'm eating a ton of corn now. I forgot to mention that. Carrots. I had some carrots. They actually taste pretty good when they're roasted in the oven, but not too soft."

"Good! Yes. And tofu can be really good. It all depends on how it's prepared. There's so much. Just keep trying new things. You'll be surprised. Go to the Asian markets. Go to the Mexican markets. There's a whole world of food out there that's just beginning to open up for you."

"Huh. Yeah. I never thought of it that way. Kind of like a new adventure, I guess."

"Very much. But also, tell me about exercise," she said. "Have you been trying to take a walk or do anything else?"

"Oh, my gosh! How could I forget to tell you! Yes! I got a dog!"

"What?" she said. She looked genuinely pleased. "You did?"

"I went to Humane Society Silicon Valley, just like you said, and they matched me with a middle-aged overweight dog so we can both try to get healthy together."

"Wow, Eric, that's fantastic! What's his name?"

"Peety."

"Peety. So, you're taking him out to walk at least twice a day?"

"Yes. We've only walked to the end of the block and back. Real slow so far. The people at the HSSV told me to take it slow with him, too. And so far so good."

"Well, I have to say, you're an excellent patient. You're off to a very good start. There are a couple of things I want to talk to you about, though. Your blood work showed some of what we expected. The diabetes. The cholesterol is extremely high. Liver function is impaired. There are indications that your digestion is not efficient, which means you're not absorbing the nutrients you need even when you eat properly. And your testosterone level is extremely low, which—"

"Really?" I said. "How low? What do you mean?"

"There are a couple of measurements we look at, but your overall level is below three hundred units, which, at your age, it should be almost double that. According to the charts, you have the testosterone of an eighty-year-old man," she said.

I was floored.

"That...wow. That kind of explains a lot," I said. "What would cause that?"

"Diet. Exercise. Like everything else. Your organs and glands and heart are so stressed, they simply aren't functioning properly. They're working much harder than they should just to keep you alive. So what I'm going to do is start you on some supplements, just to kick-start your system and help get your body functioning better. The goal will be to take you off of them once your hormones are properly balanced and your body begins to heal, which may take a matter of months, probably no more than a year. You shouldn't need to be on any supplements whatsoever once you are healthy."

At this point I was truly ready to take any advice Dr. Preeti offered and to follow it as closely as I could. I'd done some reading and read a lot of wild marketing claims about vitamins and supplements. It's an industry that is loosely regulated at best. But I trusted Dr. Preeti to choose the best supplements for me. I also liked the idea that she was already talking about getting me off of them as soon as possible. This wasn't a scheme to sell me products or get me hooked on more pills. The idea was to get my body functioning on its own, not to mask my symptoms with pharmaceuticals that I'd be dependent on for the rest of my life.

I've always had a bit of a rebellious streak. The idea of giving profits to "the man" never sat well with me. The power and wealth of the pharmaceutical industry in America bothered me deeply, and personally, especially since such a significant chunk of my paycheck went to them each month while my health seemed to get worse with every new prescription.

The way I saw things after listening to Dr. Preeti, I believed that every doctor I'd ever visited had ignored the fact that there was a war going on in my body. I wasn't sure how the war got started, or why my body was so stressed—and in the months ahead I would do a lot of thinking about that—but the fact was, my body was at war with the foods I was eating and the medications I was taking. It seemed as if all my previous doctors had just tried to prescribe medication to camouflage and lessen my symptoms—to make it seem as if the war wasn't really happening.

What Dr. Preeti wanted to help me do was to actually end the war.

I went home that night and threw two loaves of bread into a paper bag. I dropped them off at a nearby food pantry the next morning. I didn't want the temptation in my kitchen. I looked through the cabinet and threw out some old cookies that I didn't even realize I had, which were definitely not gluten-free. I threw out an open bag of chips, even though they were vegan, just because they were full of oil. I found a website listing vegan restaurants all over the country, and I bookmarked it for future reference.

That night, I cracked open my last two cans of tuna. I decided to get it over with. I decided to eat it on a salad again. Those salads were boring. Eating raw greens was not fun, or tasty, or delicious. But I was determined to do this, so I sucked it up. On this night, in addition to not wanting to mix the tuna with any mayonnaise, I decided I didn't want to drown the salad in my favorite bottled Italian dressing, either. Dr. Preeti's mention of cutting back on oils made me want to stop consuming oils altogether. Maybe that was over-the-top, but I figured I *needed* to go over the top. So I splashed the greens with some balsamic vinegar and salt and pepper, and that was it. I let the flavors of a few tomatoes and peppers and some little sprigs of crisp broccoli stand on their own. Then I put one can of tuna on top. I didn't want the second one. It seemed like too much. I opened the other can and gave it to Peety—and that got me thinking.

If I was feeling better, feeling lighter, and had lost a little weight going mostly vegan for a week, I wondered if Peety's health might improve if he went vegan, too.

I went online and looked up vegan dog foods. It turns out there were people in the pet world who swore by such a diet for their dogs. People talked about it working "miracles" for their dogs' problems, including joint and skin conditions. I found a whole bunch of veterinarians online stating that it was perfectly safe, although some said it was "unnatural" and "bad" for animals, who were meat eaters by nature. (I saw the same critiques about humans switching to vegan diets, too.) But I found the evidence arguing *for* vegan dog food to be much stronger than the evidence against. So I kept searching and found recipes for homemade dog foods, and extensive lists of all sorts of "people foods" that were healthy for dogs—as well as lists of foods that dogs should never eat, including onions, and grapes, and of course dark chocolate.

The next day I went out and bought Peety a commercially produced vegan dog food. He loved it. He gobbled it up as if it were a steak dinner.

Sally came in and cleaned the apartment again a few days later. It had only been a week, and yet she said she'd never seen so much hair from any one dog in all of her years cleaning people's homes. I apologized to her. (How embarrassing is it to have to apologize to your cleaning person for the mess your dog made?)

Three days later, I woke up in the morning and realized I had slept through the night. Peety's scratching hadn't woken me up. Not once. I worked entirely from home that day, and I kept watch over him, and I was pretty sure he didn't scratch himself at all for the rest of the day.

I couldn't help but wonder, *Did the vegan dog food alleviate his symptoms that quickly?*

Just a couple of days after that—so maybe five or six days after eliminating animal products from my diet—I woke up feeling like a new person. I stretched and rolled out of bed with ease. I stepped out of the shower and noticed there was about half as much dog hair clinging to my toes as there had been on any other day (besides the few glorious, hair-free hours on the days that Sally came). I only noticed because I could feel my feet. My ankles weren't sore. I lifted my legs and realized that my knees weren't sore, either. When I took Peety out for his morning walk, I did so in much less pain. I was still well over three hundred pounds. I still swung my legs rather than bent my knees in any sort of normal gait. I could still hear my imaginary "thump, thump, thump" when I walked. But it didn't *hurt*.

After just one week on his new diet, Peety appeared to be visibly thinner. He seemed to have a spring in his step. We walked to the end of the block and instead of turning around, we decided to keep going. We turned the corner and he led me all the way around the block. An entire city block! Peety was on patrol out in front the whole time. He still barked like crazy at other dogs who dared to cross his path, but when we passed other people, he just seemed a little less angry at the world.

It seemed like a miracle. *Was it really just the food?*

As we came upon an elderly woman sitting on her steps on the far side of the block, on a street I'd never stepped foot on before that moment despite the fact that it was the next street over, the woman spoke up: "Oh, what a cute doggie," she said.

"Thank you," I replied.

"How old is he?"

"He's about seven," I said. Peety turned and started to walk up her path.

"No, son, come on," I said.

"It's OK. Can I pet him?" she asked.

Peety seemed friendly and calm, the way he did around the employees as HSSV when we'd last stopped in. So I said, "Sure."

Peety sauntered over and let the woman scratch him behind his ears. He closed his eyes and seemed to really enjoy it.

"My father used to keep a dog like this on our farm. He would herd the sheep. He'd herd people sometimes, too," she said. "Just walk around and nudge people along until they were all standing in the same area by the barn. It was the funniest thing."

"Really? That's wild," I said.

"Do you live around here?" she asked me.

"Yes. Around the block."

"Oh. I've never seen you two before," she said.

"No, we just started taking walks together. Trying to get in shape," I said.

It was startling to have a stranger talk to me without an agenda or a reason. Strangers don't strike up conversations with solitary obese men. That's not the way the world works.

"Good for you," she said. "So I'll see you again then," she said to Peety. "What's his name?"

"Peety."

"Peety. Nice to meet you, Peety."

"Thanks," I said. I didn't even know what I was thanking her for. The word just came out of my mouth. "Come on, son."

By the time we got home, I was winded. Except for that brief chat, we hadn't stopped the whole time we were out there. I could feel my heart pounding in my chest. I was sweaty. Yet even after all of that, I didn't *hurt*.

Peety went straight for his water bowl. I went into the kitchen and drank two big glasses of water myself. I heated up some rice and beans for breakfast. I ate some fruit, including some sliced kiwi, which I tried that week for the very first time in my life. It was good!

As I sat there eating my rainbow-colored meal (which Dr. Preeti totally supported, by the way), I realized that Peety and I both felt radically different than we'd felt just a week earlier.

Not only radically different. Radically *better*.

"You feel as good as I do?" I asked him. Peety looked up at me and cocked his head to the side. His eyes seemed to almost sparkle now. He looked *so* much better, after just a week! I was shocked. I never expected a shift in a dog's diet could be so transformative.

I still questioned how much this shift in diet would accomplish for me, though. If I continued to lose weight at the rate I'd lost it the first week, that meant I was only down about ten pounds after all of this work. I wasn't sure of the number because I didn't keep a scale at home. Most home scales don't go above three hundred pounds, and who wants to look at that number on a daily basis? What's the point? To remind you of how terrible your life is?

Five pounds a week felt like awfully slow progress to me after making such a big change. But then, seeing Peety look and feel so much better gave me encouragement. The way I figured, a dog's life is supposed to be seven years for every human year. Did that mean the effects of his change to a plant-based diet were showing up seven times faster than they would show up with me?

*What will I feel like in another seven weeks?* I wondered.

I saw absolutely no reason to fight it. This was *working*.

So that very morning, I swore to myself that we were both all-in. No more meat for Peety, and no more meat for me. No more cheats. Our old ways were in the past—just like Peety's scratching and flaky skin.

I was desperate to get back to Dr. Preeti and learn more. If eliminating oils would make me feel even better, then I wanted to learn how to do that. If cutting sugar would make me feel better, then I wanted to learn how to do that, too.

## chapter 7

# Peety Takes the Lead

A few days later, I went to take Peety for his morning walk and he backed right out of his collar. He'd lost so much weight that it slipped right off of his neck and over his head. I had to tighten it two notches just to make it stay on.

After my shower that morning, I realized that my pants were almost falling off of me, too. I tightened my belt as far as it would go, but I realized that with a giant belly like mine, if my belt were to slip, then my pants would fall all the way to the floor in one swoop. That would not bode well in the middle of an appliance store.

I realized I needed to go shopping. *Clothes* shopping—an activity I hated even more than going to the grocery store.

There once was a time when I loved shopping for clothes. Especially back in the 1980s when I lived in San Francisco. That's when I discovered Nordstrom, a store that offered a high-end, premium clothes-shopping experience unlike anything I had ever encountered. At most stores I had ever shopped, the salespeople were underpaid and had terrible attitudes. It always seemed like they couldn't care less about actually helping customers. But at Nordstrom, there was always some athletic-looking sales associate ready to help find clothes that fit your needs, fit your body, and actually made you look good. They were well trained. They knew what they were doing. They knew their inventory. They talked to you and asked questions to figure out what you were looking for and how they could help. Nordstrom even gave me my first credit card. I always left that store feeling and looking like royalty, or maybe a movie star. Truly. I loved it.

Then one day, shortly after my fortieth birthday, as I was approaching 250 pounds, I walked into Nordstrom to shop for new pants. I'd gained weight quickly that year, and my pants had grown so tight I felt like a hundred pounds of potatoes in an eighty-pound sack.

I walked into the men's section and approached a model-looking salesman. I asked him if he could help me.

The man gave me an odd look. He then encircled the circumference of my stomach with a cloth measuring tape and said, "I'm sorry, you'll need to go to a big-and-tall store. We don't carry above a forty-two-inch waist."

I couldn't believe it. He completely dismissed me and then turned around to start talking to somebody else.

I felt humiliated.

I suppose someone else might have taken that as their rock bottom, in-the-gutter moment. I wished I had done that. Instead, it was only the beginning of my transformation into a man with an apple-shaped body and toothpick legs. It would take me another ten years, an additional one hundred pounds, and ten more inches of waist size before I would hit my bottom and cause a whole plane full of people to get delayed.

My favorite store abandoned me, and so I walked into a Men's Wearhouse—which was a very different experience from Nordstrom. I quickly discovered that quality clothing and fashion does not exist for obese men. There has been some improvement since that time, but for the most part, the majority of what's available for men over three hundred pounds is the equivalent of a muumuu: low-end, loud, Hawaiian-print shirts.

The fact is, most fashion designers want to design clothes that look good on people, and they don't want people who *don't* look good in their clothes to wear their label in public.

And so I avoided shopping. For years.

Now? I had no choice. I couldn't have my pants falling down. So I trekked to Ross and Marshalls, hoping to spend as little money as possible and get out as fast as I could. I would have ordered clothes online if I could have, but I didn't know what size I was anymore. My size varied wildly between 2XL and 4XL depending on the particular brand, and after losing a couple of inches, I definitely had to try everything on.

The bending and squatting of dressing and undressing in tiny dressing rooms left me overheated and miserable. This was not a fun shopping spree for my new slightly smaller self. This wasn't a triumph. It wasn't a victory lap. It was awful. I hated being surrounded by mirrors. I wanted to black them out. Being forced to look at what I'd become in the brutal sharp glare of those fluorescent lights disgusted me. I felt angrier than ever that I had allowed myself to get so fat in the first place.

I bought three new pair of pants, and a few new shirts, and spent nearly two hundred dollars. It felt like a rip-off. The clothing felt cheap. The fabrics didn't breathe. I knew I would sweat every time I wore them. But I had no choice.

After ringing me up, the rail-thin girl behind the counter said, "Have a nice day."

I wanted to tell her to go eat a pizza.

I went home, and sitting on the couch that night I thought maybe I should give it all up. Maybe it just wasn't worth it. Maybe I was too far-gone.

Then Peety jumped into my lap. Out of nowhere and for no reason whatsoever, he careened up onto the couch and landed right on me. He started licking my face, which made me laugh, and I petted him.

"What are you doing, boy?"

He pressed himself into my belly and lay down on the top of my thick thighs as if he were a tiny puppy snuggling up in a blanket.

And then he looked up at me as if I were the greatest guy in the world.

"Oh, Peety," I said. "Are you sure you're not disappointed you wound up with me?"

He kept looking at me with those beautiful dark eyes. I'd heard people talk about dogs smiling before, and I thought they were nuts. I thought they were just projecting. But all of a sudden, Peety smiled. He opened his teeth slightly and pulled up the corners of his mouth. My boy was smiling! It was unbelievable. Suddenly I was no longer feeling sorry for myself but instead was thinking about Peety's happiness.

I stopped petting him for a second to stare at his beautiful face, and he immediately nudged my hand, urging me to get back to it.

"OK!" I said. "That better?"

As I continued to pet him, he squinted his eyes and kept smiling, clearly enjoying the simple pleasure of my hand stroking the back of his neck.

"I'm sorry, son," I said. "I don't mean to get down. I'll try harder, OK? I promise I won't let you down."

Six weeks later, Peety looked like a brand-new dog. A month and a half into his new vegan diet, having made no other changes, Peety was approaching an ideal weight for a dog of his size and build. He was no longer lethargic. In fact, I would say he was downright energetic. He had no more skin problems. None. He was still a shedder, but the over-shedding, the piling up of hair tumbleweeds all over the apartment within hours, ceased. Best of all, his eyes had a twinkle the likes of which I'd never seen.

When I uttered the words, "Want to go for a walk?" Peety no longer sauntered to the door. He jumped up, ran to the door, and did circles around and around until I managed to get his leash hooked on. He'd pull me down the hall to the elevator and pull me out at the bottom floor. Every time.

I'd finally managed to train him to wait to go pee on the grass, too. I had learned some positive-reinforcement training techniques, which worked by praising and giving him training treats for good behavior. But the main reason for this milestone was because I could move better myself. After six weeks of plant-based eating, when we exited the elevator I could do so at a slight jog. So I started running as soon as the doors opened, all the way past the concrete entryway and onto the grass before he had a chance to lift a leg.

Once he got used to it, I didn't have to trick him anymore—he began associating grass with going to the bathroom and stopped peeing on the cement.

I tried to take Peety to the obedience classes HSSV had asked me to take him to when I adopted him, but it just didn't work. All of those other dogs on leashes set him off. He wouldn't stop barking and tugging on the leash. Neither he nor I liked the sounds of the clickers they used as a training method in the first class, either. I'm sure it works for other dogs, but it seemed to stress him out, which stressed *me* out. So I gave up after two classes. The way I saw it, Peety had endured enough stress for one lifetime. I didn't need to add new stress to his life. I felt my job was to take his stress away. So I decided to simply let Peety be Peety. Plus, he kept improving and getting better all on his own. He grew friendlier and friendlier with every pound he lost. When we took walks, he was still "leash reactive," but he didn't keep his haunches up all the time. He still patrolled the sidewalks, keeping watch over his fiefdom as he guarded our block, but his whole demeanor became much more approachable. He seemed to look forward to seeing that old lady on the steps when she was there, and more and more people stopped to pet him on a fairly regular basis.

I'll never forget the first time an attractive, thirty-something woman stopped us on the corner. "What a cute dog," she said.

"Thanks," I said to her. And she *smiled*.

What was really remarkable was how often those same people struck up a conversation with me while they petted my dog.

"How old is he?" they might ask. Or, "What kind of a dog is he?" And that would lead to them sharing some story about their own dog, or the dog they had when they were a kid, and sometimes that would lead to a discussion of the weather, or something that was going on in the news.

Peety's weight loss, and his change in demeanor, almost magically made *me* less invisible.

Back on our very first walk together, I told Peety to go ahead and take the lead, and he did. Once he started feeling better, he led me not only around the block, but sometimes around the block again. One day, he turned left instead of right and we walked around the next block, and then back across in front of our building and around our block in one giant figure eight. He followed the very same route that night and the next morning. And then the next day he got to the end of the second block and wanted to keep going. So I tagged along. We covered nearly four blocks that day, and he marked his way on various trees and fence posts as we went. It's as if he were mapping out his neighborhood and claiming new territory for himself every few days.

Over the course of those weeks, Peety kept pulling harder and harder on the leash, raring to go, and there were times when I simply could not keep up, even though I'd dropped five pounds a week pretty consistently since I started plant-based eating and walking. I was about to break the three-hundred-pound barrier I hadn't broken in years. I'd expanded my tastes and cooking abilities. I even tackled tofu, which I was wrong to judge as nothing more than a tasteless slimy white block of slop that even the army wouldn't serve. I realized after some trial and error that it was an incredibly nutritious and versatile food. I managed to sauté cubes of tofu and incorporate it into a stir-fry that I actually enjoyed eating. I'd stocked up on more spices than I ever knew existed and was quickly learning how to use them. By avoiding bread and processed foods, the misery of headaches, abdominal pain, and overall discomfort disappeared.

I felt good. Not just better, but really *good*.

Still, I'd done some more reading about herding dogs at that point, and it seemed obvious to me that I wasn't giving Peety enough room to roam. Now that he was feeling good, he was clearly itching to run. It was just in his nature. These were dogs bred for covering miles and miles of fields, running back and forth, herding sheep or goats or cows for hours on end every day of their lives. Even if Peety didn't have all of that in him, I imagined he had more of it than I was allowing him to express on the end of a leash on hard concrete sidewalks.

He and I shared a home. We slept in the same bed. We spent every morning and evening together, as well as whole days side-by-side whenever I worked from home, which was often. I think it's safe to say we were "bonding"—even though I was starting to realize that I barely knew what that word meant.

Watching his transformation over those six weeks only inspired me to want to do more for him. When I looked into his eyes, I knew I wanted Peety to have the best life he could. I wanted him to enjoy himself. I wanted to help make up for the crappy life of abandonment and lousy food and pain and suffering he'd endured for far too long.

So I started to take him places with me. He finally figured out how to jump into the backseat, and he lay down back there most of the time while I drove. He seemed very content hunkered down in that seat for some reason. It was still winter, so it wasn't scorching hot in San Jose, which meant I could leave him in the car, in the shade, with the windows cracked open for short periods of time while I ran into a store, or even when I stopped in to say hello to clients, as long as I knew those meetings wouldn't last long.

I decided to take him into Petco with me one day, and it was the weirdest thing. Just like he'd done at the HSSV store, Peety didn't bark or get upset at any of the other dogs he encountered as we walked those aisles. Outside in the parking lot, he barked up an angry storm at every dog he saw. But inside the store, he walked right by them with a quick sniff and a look as if he were tipping his hat in a sort of friendly hello. It reminded me of that old *Road Runner Show* cartoon, where the sheepdog and Wile E. Coyote were at each other's throats all day, but then they clocked out, as if they were ending their shifts, and they started talking to each other like normal people—as if they were only mortal enemies when they were on the clock.

Outdoors was the place where Peety worked. In stores, he was off the clock.

Still, I wanted to do more for him. So I went online and

looked around to see what sorts of parks I could find in our area.

Lo and behold, when I opened Google maps I noticed a great big park just up the street from where we lived. It was only about a mile away. It looked huge! You could only see a little corner of it from the road. I'd driven past it dozens of times, maybe hundreds of times, but I'd never stopped. I never knew that park had a name. I had noticed its tree-lined paths, busy with runners and walkers, some even walking dogs, but to me, for as long as I'd lived there, it had just been a fleeting landmark on my way to someplace else. I had no idea what treasures that park might hold beyond the open green spaces I could see from my car window.

For Peety's sake, I thought it was time we find out.

## chapter 8

# Oh, the Water...

 What do you think, boy? Wanna try someplace new today?"

Peety stopped and looked up at me with his eyes all wide.
Everything about him shouted, "Yes, yes, yes!" He wasn't
just wagging his tail. He was wagging his whole rear end.

"OK, OK," I said. "Sit, boy. Sit. Let me get your leash
on."

The farthest we'd gone to the north of us was McKee
Road. We'd usually turn one way or the other and circle back
around. We'd gone the other way and walked past the store-
fronts and turned left on Alum Rock Avenue to go watch the
cars zoom by from the I-680 overpass. But I felt that Peety
needed a destination. Someplace with a payoff. Someplace
where he could let loose and be a dog.

"I think you're gonna like this," I said to him as we passed
McKee and kept on walking northwest past Independence
High School.

From my research, I knew there were certain city parks

that didn't allow dogs at all, which surprised me, but there were also plenty that did—most marked by strict rules about picking up after your pet and keeping dogs on leash. Those rules made sense to me. I mean, who wants to have their kids walking around doggie land mines, or have strange dogs running up to them while they're trying to enjoy a day in the park? I didn't plan to let Peety off leash anyway. The idea that he might run away or get hit by a car was terrifying to me.

As far as I knew, Peety had never been off leash except in the confines of our condo, a kennel, or someone's fenced-in backyard. So I had no idea what would happen if he suddenly had that kind of freedom.

The thing I noticed about this particular park, though, other than its location just over one mile from our condo, was that according to the website, Penitencia Creek County Park was home to a stunning pond full of ducks and wildlife. The photos I found were beautiful, showing birds on that water with the golden mountains off in the background, like something out of *National Geographic*.

*How could something like that exist so close to where I live and I not even know it's there?*

As soon as I saw that picture I wondered something else, too: *I wonder if Peety would like to go for a swim?*

That's exactly what I planned to find out on this hot afternoon.

"Peety, heel!" I said.

He never heeled. I'm not sure why I kept saying it every day, but I did.

"Heel. Heel!" From the moment we passed the high

school and caught a glimpse of the park entrance, he kept choking himself at the end of the leash trying to run ahead. It's as if he'd Googled it on his own and knew exactly where we were headed. "Will you just hold on, boy," I said. I'd never seen him like this. It cracked me up. "Peety, son! Hold on!" I shouted.

I picked up my pace as best I could, trying to give him a little slack on the leash as we turned off the sidewalk and headed down a path that I hoped would lead to the pond. Peety glanced at a few squirrels running across the lawn and tipped his ears up to the chirping birds in the trees, but I swear he was on a mission. He just kept pulling forward, panting as he pulled.

Then all of a sudden, he stopped. He cocked his head to the side.

He heard something.

"What is it, boy?" I whispered.

I squatted down as best I could to try to hear what he heard. I stopped breathing for a few seconds just to listen— and I heard it. It wasn't much more than a murmur. I might have missed it if I'd kept crunching my sneakers on the gravelly path. But as soon as I stopped and listened, like Peety, I heard it clear as day: the distant quacking of ducks. Lots and lots of ducks.

"You want to go see 'em?" I said. Peety lurched forward.

I couldn't run to save my life, but I tried to keep up with him, all hobbling and awkward as he yanked on the leash.

"Man, you really want to see those ducks!" I puffed, laughing and trying to catch my breath.

Suddenly there it was, recessed deep in the lush greenery,

glistening in the late-afternoon sun just twenty yards ahead of us: a beautiful pond teeming with waterfowl. There must have been a hundred birds on that water.

"Acchhh-aacchhh-aacchhh," Peety hacked, pulling so hard on the leash he could barely breathe.

"Stop it, boy," I said. "Sit, now. Sit."

He sat and I petted him behind the ears. "Have you ever gone swimming before?" I asked him. I had never understood why people talked to their dogs. But clearly, dogs listen. And often, they answer. In a look, a bark, a whimper, a tip of the head—they *answer*.

What I picked up from Peety in that moment didn't make clear to me if he'd ever seen a big body of water before in his life, let alone gone swimming. What he did make clear, though, is that he wanted to get into that water *right now*.

As I squatted there, holding his collar, holding him back, the thought of keeping that grip on him suddenly bothered me. *Aren't dogs meant to run?* I thought. *Aren't they built for it? Isn't that just part of what they do?* I thought about the notion that Peety's whole life had been lived either pent up, caged up, or tied to the end of a leash, and I suddenly saw it from a new perspective—not my selfish, parent-like worrying perspective that he might run off or get hurt if I let him off leash, but from his point of view instead. What kind of a life was that? The fact that he was so overweight and hurting so much until just these last few weeks meant he had been living in a cage of a different kind, too.

*How could anyone allow a dog to get so out of shape that he didn't even want to run?*

Changing Peety's diet and taking these walks had freed

him. Maybe it was time to let him experience what freedom really feels like.

I looked around and there were hardly any people in the vicinity of the pond. So I didn't think twice about whether he might run off or bother anyone else in the park. I knew he was laser focused on that water.

"You want to get in that pond, don't you, boy?" I said.

Holding his collar tightly in my left hand, I quietly, carefully unhooked the leash with my right. The tiny "click" of the clip unlatching made his ears perk up. He stopped his panting and looked at me, making sure he heard what he thought he heard.

"Be careful now, OK?" I said.

Peety licked my cheek in a flurry of kisses, and I knew this was the right thing to do.

"OK, boy," I whispered. "Go on!"

I let go of his collar and Peety took off like a sprinter at the Olympics: head down, body forward, legs moving so fast they almost overtook him. I couldn't believe how quickly he ran. He flew down the path and didn't slow down one bit as he approached the water's edge. Instead, when he got to the water, he *leaped*. My jaw dropped open as he sailed out over the pond. He must've traveled seven feet through the air before he landed in a great big belly flop. The tremendous sound of it caused every head to turn and look our way, and the splash sent every duck and other bird in that pond up into the air all at once. In a single second the sky filled with all of those birds, quacking and screeching in a giant, swarming mosaic silhouetted against the pale late-afternoon sun.

I realized later that letting a dog off leash like that in a public place was a naive and potentially dangerous thing to do. A lot of other dogs might have taken off and kept on running until they were good and lost. I'm just glad that wasn't the case with Peety. His natural instincts as a herder, I think, are what led him to stick close by me.

Nonetheless, I hurried to the pond's edge to make sure Peety was OK. I sure hoped he wasn't drowning or anything, because I'm not sure if I could have swum far enough to go rescue him. I got to the edge and there he was, swimming in circles like a champ.

He was free.

Peety swam so hard he practically lifted his whole front end right out of the water, beaming with pride and excitement.

"Good job!" I yelled. "Woo-hoo!"

When he heard me he swam to shore, ran out of the water, beelined it right up to me, and launched into a reverberating full-body shake of biblical proportions. He completely drenched me with mud and pond water, and not for one second did it make me angry. In fact, I laughed. I loved it. And in that moment, I realized I loved *him*.

*I love this dog!*

I loved having this dog. I loved caring for this dog. I loved everything about this moment. I didn't even realize how hot I was until Peety ran up and cooled me off, and then I wasn't worried about getting dirty, or getting wet. All of that stuff that we humans worry about all the time—looking good for others, being neat and proper—all of it seemed to fade away.

I was still laughing as he turned around and ran back into the water for another swim.

Most of the birds seemed to settle down on the far side of the pond pretty quickly. I think they figured out that Peety wasn't interested in hurting any of them. He just wanted to get into that water and maybe see what they were up to. I hoped no one else in the park minded that he was off leash and swimming, but frankly, I could not have cared less if they did. If a cop or a park ranger wandered by and wanted to fine me for it, I would have gladly paid the ticket. Watching my boy enjoy himself in this moment of pure doggy bliss was worth any price.

Peety did the swim-to-shore, shake-off, and run-back-into-the-water thing about eight more times before I was able to get him to sit and rest for a minute. He was panting like crazy, but between the sparkle in his eyes and the sight of his tongue hanging out of his big doggy smile I knew he was perfectly OK.

Once again, he looked up at me like I was the greatest guy in the world—and that is exactly what I wanted to be for him. I wanted to fulfill Peety's every dream. And in that moment, I felt like the two of us could have done anything.

"Want to keep walking?" I asked him.

Peety stood right up and circled around as if we were still at the door back home, raring to go as if the mile-plus we'd already walked and all of that swimming hadn't taken a thing out of him.

The path we were on seemed to go all the way out around the perimeter of the park in one big loop. I guessed it was at least a half-mile around, and yet for some reason it didn't seem daunting to me. I guess I was raring to go, too.

I clipped Peety back on leash and said, "OK, boy. Let's do this."

Peety dripped a trail of water as we walked, and I couldn't help but smile at the bounce in his step. I wouldn't have described his walk as slow and plodding back when we first started walking together, but I could tell now that it clearly was. In fact, we both seemed to be moving at a much better clip together. We didn't jog or run-walk or move anywhere close to a pace that someone would call "fast," but the occasional pedestrians who passed us on the sidewalk no longer flew by us like we were stuck in the breakdown lane with our flashers on, either.

We managed to make it all the way to the far side of the pond in a matter of minutes. And maybe it's just because I was all wet from Peety's shaking, but I didn't even break a sweat as we walked. It was just incredible to me. I was down thirty pounds, and I felt like a different human being. And even after all of that swimming, Peety was still walking ahead of me, leading me on, with no signs of slowing down.

My knees hurt by the time we came back around to the spot where Peety had jumped in, though, and I wondered if his hurt, too. I had to remember that I was still a three-hundred-pound man. And Peety wasn't a puppy. Carrying all that weight around had to have taken a toll on him, too. I worried for a moment that maybe we'd both been overly ambitious. The prior week I'd picked up a Garmin GPS watch to try to keep track of how much distance we were covering in our daily walks, and my estimate was correct. According to my watch, that loop around the park was .6 of a mile. It was definitely going to hurt to make a 1.2-mile walk back home after going that extra distance. By the time we were home we'd have walked nearly three miles in a single afternoon.

"*Three miles!*" I said. "Peety, that's huge!"

A mere two months earlier even the *thought* of walking three miles seemed too painful to bear. I never could have done it, even if my life depended on it. I'm sure of it. I would have collapsed.

How had I gone from being in that state to now willingly walking 1.2 miles to a park, and then *wanting* to walk an additional .6-mile loop around a pond just—for what? For *fun*? Is that what this was? I wasn't sure I had ever gone out of my way to walk for fun in my whole life. Why did I want to do it now?

The reason was panting at my feet.

I thought about the aches and pains I felt—actually stopped and thought about them—and I realized they were nothing compared to the way I felt just walking from the bedroom to the bathroom on any given day before I met Peety.

We stopped for a minute to catch our breath, and Peety sat with his head leaned up against my achy right knee. We looked out at those ducks together, and he kept looking up at me with the biggest smile, his tongue bright pink as he panted and begged me with his eyes for another swim.

"Not today, son," I said. "You just dried off."

"Woof!" he barked.

"I know, I know. But you must be hungry. I know I am. We'll come back this weekend, I promise. OK?"

"Woof!" he barked again. Only this time, he got up, took one last look at those ducks on the pond, then turned around and started walking toward home. He instinctively knew which way to go. So I once again let Peety take the lead— this time for a long, achy, wonderful walk back home.

We'd made a habit of taking our morning and evening walks before breakfast and dinner, respectively, which yielded an unexpected benefit: there was something about all of that movement and expending of energy before I ate that made me feel full faster. It's the complete opposite of what I would have expected, but the effect was consistently noticeable. Getting that exercise made me less hungry.

I took Peety out one last time before bed most nights, too, so he could go to the bathroom, and we'd often walk all the way to the end of the block. Just because. We didn't give it a thought. It was astounding to me how much shorter that block now seemed.

On that particular night after our extra-long walk to the park, I made a double-size tofu stir-fry with no onions so that Peety and I could share it. I put it on two nice plates and we sat together on the floor of the living room and shared that delicious meal.

"We ought to do this more often," I said to him.

The fact that I could sit on the floor with my back against the sofa was pretty astounding. Since my knees hurt from the distance we'd traveled, I worried I might have trouble getting up, but a couple of months earlier I never would have *attempted* to sit on that floor. For years I didn't bend or squat or put my body in any position other than standing, sit-ting, or lying down unless it was absolutely necessary.

*Just how caged up had I been?*

I felt a sort of buzz as I sat on that floor, almost as if I'd downed a few shots of espresso. My knees hurt, and I was tired from the long walk, but I felt energized at the same time.

From my new vantage point, I looked around my condo. I had referred to it as "my apartment" at times, but it wasn't an apartment. It wasn't a rental. I owned it. I could do almost anything I wanted to it. Yet in all the time since I'd purchased it, I'd done nothing. The space was sparsely furnished with the sorts of things you'd expect to find in a bachelor pad after college: a glass-top coffee table, a small table with two chairs in the kitchen, a basic sofa, and a really big flat-screen TV. The walls were white. My dining room table was covered with work-related files and boxes. The spare bedroom had a bed and nightstand, and nothing else. My own bedroom had a king-size bed on a basic frame, with no headboard.

I looked around and realized I was living in a plain white box.

"You know," I said to Peety, "maybe we ought to fix this place up."

# chapter 9

# Rebuilding

I let the thought go. I got busy with work. The post-exercise energy buzz didn't last.

As an obese person, you get used to not doing things. Especially for yourself. The choice to say no is easier than the choice to get motivated, because getting motivated usually involves pain. In fact, once that mentality sets in, shedding the mental sloth is tougher than the physical act of losing the weight.

I did manage to stay focused on Peety, though, and the quest to find new walking destinations in order to make his life more complete. We made it back to the pond on Saturday, just like I promised, and once again Peety ran and jumped and splashed in multiple moments of pure glory. But the following weekend, we decided to walk an equivalent distance in the opposite direction. We crossed the I-680 overpass, which is as far as we'd ever gone along Alum Rock Avenue, and we kept going. In a car, if we had zoomed right through and kept going for a few miles, we would have climbed into the hills and wound up at Mount Hamilton, with the University of California observatory that proved Einstein's theory of relativity. I'd driven through that area quite a few times. But in a car, I never noticed this one little block, almost like a little town center that you'd find in some small town; a blast-from-the-past full of mom-and-pop shops on both sides of the street.

The first place that caught my eye was Mario's Barber Shop. I was in need of a haircut, and though I normally tried to get that experience over with as fast as I could by going to some hair-cutting chain, I thought to myself, *Why not?*

I opened the door next to the swirling old-fashioned barbershop sign, and a little bell chimed. I felt like I was walking back in time. I half expected to see a man from a Norman Rockwell painting with a handlebar mustache cutting hair in a white smock. Instead, I caught my first glimpse of Mario: a Mexican barber whose stomach was bigger around than mine was at its peak, and whose personality was even bigger than that. There were five or six guys sitting in red-vinyl-upholstered chairs along the wall, and they all looked up to see who'd stepped into their world. I immediately felt like I was walking into an exclusive club, where I wasn't quite sure I'd be welcomed. As a white guy in that neighborhood, I was definitely the odd man out in this particular room.

"Hey! Does your pup want a haircut?" Mario asked loudly. Everyone laughed.

"No, but I do. Can you fit me in?"

He was just wrapping up one man's haircut, and a man in the chair closest to him stood up.

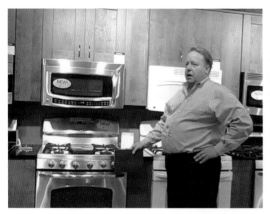

Eric's "before" photo from 2010 at 340 pounds, the day before the airplane flight that changed everything.

Eric's "after" photo one year later in 2011, feeling confident and happy at the gym.

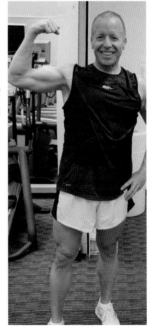

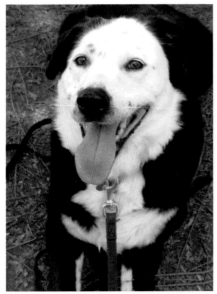

Peety looking happy and feeling proud at Penitencia Creek Park after drying off from jumping into the duck pond.

Peety modeling next to furniture Eric reupholstered to match Peety's fur, at their condo in San Jose, California.

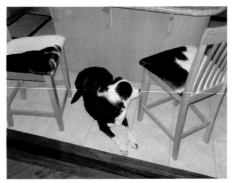

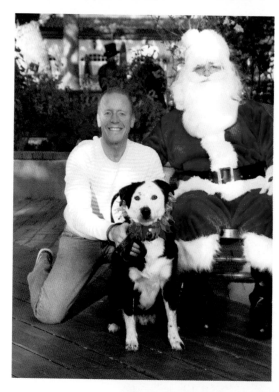

Eric and Peety at Humane Society Silicon Valley's 2012 annual Santa event for adopted pets in Los Gatos, California.

Eric and Peety sharing a hug at one of Eric's dinner party fund-raisers in 2012 (photo credit Michele Taylor Cehn).

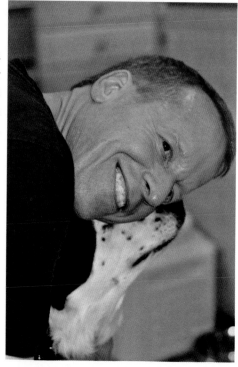

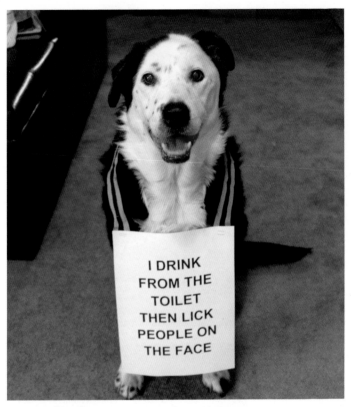

Peety and his fair-warning sign from 2013.

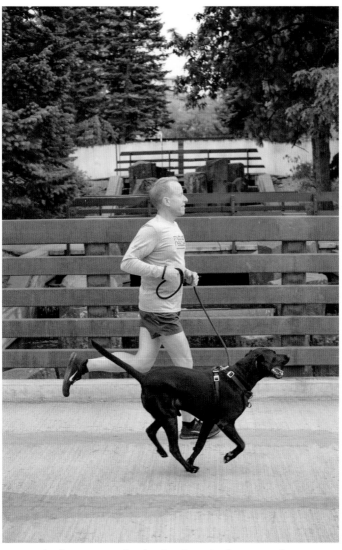

Eric and Jake running for the finish in Spokane, Washington, in 2016 (photo credit Vanessa Mathisen).

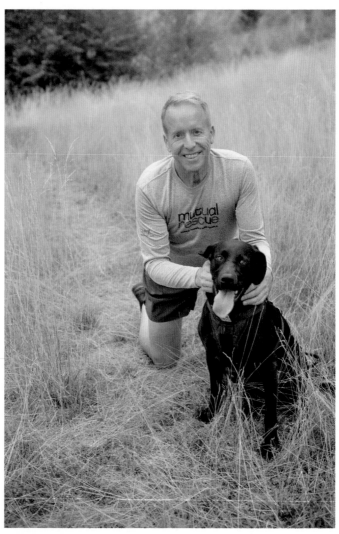

Eric and Jake posing for a magazine cover, 2016 (photo credit
Vanessa Mathisen).

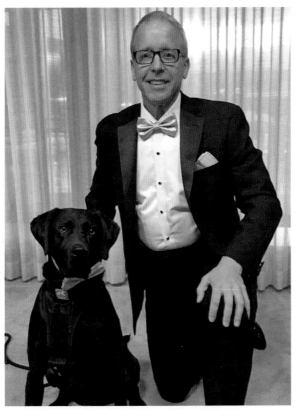

Eric and Jake at the Seattle Humane Tuxes and Tails event in Bellevue, Washington, in 2016, where they walked the runway.

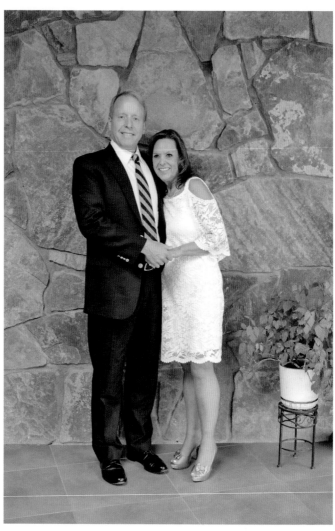

Eric and Jaye's wedding photo in 2017 at St. Mary's Church in Spokane Valley, Washington (photo credit Vanessa Mathisen).

"Sure. Have a seat," Mario said.

"Come on, boy," I said to Peety, and I walked toward the just-vacated chair, only to get a whole room full of stares. The guy in the adjacent seat said a few terse words in Spanish that I couldn't understand, but I quickly realized that I had broken protocol. I was supposed to take the chair closest to the door. Whenever a haircut was completed, everyone would move down one seat until they were next in line.

"Oh, sorry. Sorry," I said as I shuffled Peety back toward the chair by the door.

Peety lay right down on the cool, black-and-white-tile floor and seemed perfectly content as we waited. I took that as a good sign that I was right where I was supposed to be.

"You're new here," Mario said to me.

"Yeah, I was just out taking Peety here for a walk, and I'd never been on this block before."

"Well, you found the right place," Mario said. "Best haircut in town. I guarantee it. Just ask any lady you see. Every lady loves the man with one of Mario's haircuts!"

"Really," I said.

"It's true," he said. "Because all the ladies love Mario!"

"Wow," I said as the crew of waiting customers all chuckled. "I can't wait."

It was just so strange to walk into a place and have anyone start joking around with me. It's as if the presence of that dog opened a magical door that allowed people to see me as a human being, and not just some fat guy. Granted, Mario was significantly larger than me, so maybe he just looked at me as the same as everyone else. But I was starting to notice that in most instances, no matter where I went, people tended to speak about the dog first, if not speak *to* the dog first.

After years of suffering the loneliness of the nearly universal silent treatment from strangers, I sure welcomed the icebreaker Peety provided.

As I sat there watching customers full of lively, half-understandable conversations come and go, long before I even sat in his chair, I knew that Mario would be my go-to barber from that moment forward. Turns out he really did give a great haircut. And on a Saturday morning filled with laughter and boasts from this giant of a man who truly believed he was God's gift to women, the experience was something far more than just a haircut.

Once we became regulars, Mario would always have a treat for Peety. It's almost as if he knew how to figure out whatever a person, or dog, needed in order to keep them coming back. In the months ahead, a series of competitors would open barbershops right across the street, trying to capitalize on Mario's popularity by selling haircuts for $10, and even $6 compared to Mario's premium price of $20 per cut. But those other shops all soon went out of business. Mario's customers were too loyal, and his personality and his skills were too great. His business just kept on thriving.

He called it his one-man-union barbershop. His Teamster placard was posted on the wall of his shop. He paid his dues, he was his own manager, and man oh man was he proud of his operation.

That morning when I walked out with my first Mario haircut, Peety and I both noticed a little shop tucked almost behind Mario's, down a little driveway that kept it nearly hidden from view from the street. The awning had Chinese writing on it, and I thought it looked a little out of place in what was clearly a Mexican neighborhood. But then I noticed a green neon sign in the window that said "Grooming."

"Hey, maybe you can get a haircut, too, Peety!" I said.

Sure enough, it was a pet-grooming business, and it, too, felt like a blast-from-the-past. The shop wasn't all neat and clean like some generic, big-box pet-store grooming facility. To this day, I don't even know if that shop has a name. But the people behind the counter were friendly as could be, and they promised to get Peety all cleaned and brushed and feeling like new, so I let them get to work. Sure enough, Peety walked out looking like he'd gone on a weeklong spa vacation. He was as handsome as I'd ever seen him.

Before long, we were making walks to that little neighborhood every weekend. Because they recognized Peety, the shop owners would always wave and say hello to us. I started using a dry cleaner on that block, dropping my shirts off during the week and picking them up on our walks. As my ankle swelling and foot pain disappeared with the weight loss, I bought a pair of cowboy boots from El Rodeo Menswear on the corner. I didn't have much of an occasion to wear them, but it sure felt great to step into a pair of shoes that were fun, different, and not specifically designed for obese feet. And it felt great to support all of those little independent stores.

Mario was what I would call an expert eater, and he told me about all sorts of great hole-in-the-wall Mexican restaurants. I found that almost any of them were willing to cook me up a meat-and-cheese-free concoction, usually with fresh-grilled veggies they'd just purchased at the market that morning, popped into a corn tortilla with some *pico de gallo* and hot sauce. It was the perfect lunch and so incredibly delicious that I didn't miss the usual meat-and-cheese staples of Mexican food for one second.

One of the really incredible things about switching to a plant-based diet was that my tastes started to change after only a couple of months. The more often I used exotic spices to add flavor to what would have been a bland rice-and-beans dish, the more my taste buds started to crave those bolder flavors. I had never been a fan of spicy food in my life; yet after the first two months I started using all sorts of hot sauces on my food. Especially in restaurants. It turned out there were more vegan options available in many international-food restaurants than you'd find in the typical American joint. Tofu and various beans and vegetarian fare are staples in most Asian countries. But in order to stick to my plant-only intentions, I'd have to learn to ask certain questions, like whether they boiled their rice in chicken broth, or to please leave out the fish sauce. After a little trial and error I learned how to ask those questions and get the results I needed with hardly a hesitation. And it was in those restaurants where I quickly went from ordering my dishes mild, then medium, then hot, then extra hot. When waiters or waitresses at Mexican, Thai, or Indian restaurants gave me a scale of hot from one to five, I started choosing five. They would always try to dissuade me. Their eyes would get real wide. "Are you sure? That's really hot!" they would say. I had more than one waiter point out the fact that I was a "white guy," and that most "white guys" can't handle the hottest level of spice. It wasn't a racist thing. They were genuinely concerned that I would get sick in their restaurant, or maybe run screaming for a water pitcher, or maybe just complain and send the food back. It wasn't the norm for them to see someone who could have passed for the Pillsbury Doughboy order anything higher than a three. But I'd always go for it, and I'd always enjoy the result.

There was an added benefit to eating hot-and-spicy meals, too: the spice from peppers has been shown to increase metabolism, which meant that every time I added that great flavor and heat, I was also burning more calories.

Dr. Preeti talked with me a lot about that change in palate.

"The first phase of getting healthy is really about retraining your taste buds and increasing nutrient-dense foods in your diet. That's why we are not counting calories but simply increasing fruits and vegetables while eliminating meat, dairy, animal products, plus anything you may have a sensitivity to. Cutting calories is not our first concern. Our concern revolves around making sure that you have optimal digestion, absorption, and metabolism, which are essential for healthy and sustainable weight loss. The second phase, then, is trying to learn how to incorporate these healthier food options on a regular basis, to make them a habit, to help your body sustain optimal health," she told me. "That second phase is when we start cutting out the oils, some fats, eating less sugar, and eating fewer and fewer processed foods. That automatically reduces your calorie intake, so you don't really have to think about calories then, either."

I was surprised to learn that some people gain a lot of weight after going vegan. They eat a diet that consists mostly of what I refer to as "vegan junk food," the plethora of prepackaged meals and protein bars and desserts that have no animal product in them, but which are high in calories and fats and oils that don't necessarily contribute to a healthy lifestyle.

Even if it's not the prepackaged stuff, the added calories that go into frying and sautéing, even stir-frying with various vegetable oils, can increase the calories in a meal by one-third or more.

I knew I didn't want to make this shift only to start putting weight back on. The weight loss I'd experienced so far felt miraculously easy. My walks with Peety had turned into mini-adventures that simply made my life more interesting and interactive with the world, and the foods I ate were more delicious than most foods I'd ever eaten in my life. Plus, I ate as much as I wanted. I could eat until I felt full, and yet I no longer got tired and felt like napping after every meal. On a daily basis I woke up in the morning after a good night's sleep and felt ready to stand up and start my day. And I did so with less and less pain every week.

The more the pain went away, the easier it was to move. The more I moved, the better I felt. The better I felt, the easier it became to put in the effort. I wanted to get out more, for Peety's sake.

It's funny all the things you notice when you're out walking a dog. Beyond discovering Mario's and adding that new little town center to my life, I noticed a vibrancy and uniqueness in the Mexican community around me that had truly been invisible to me before. From the colors and furnishings in the restaurants and shops, to the overall importance of *fa-*

*milia.* For instance, every weekend there were car washes going on in one empty parking lot or another in that neighborhood. What I never knew until I went walking by with Peety is that those car washes were *funeral* car washes. Extended family members who'd lost a loved one would gather in this sort of ad hoc way out on the corner, waving cars in, trying to collect $10 per vehicle to help cover their loved one's funeral expenses. I had never seen or heard of such a thing before, in any community, in any part of the country. I admired the effort and supportive nature of it all.

Peety and I also discovered another park that week of my first Mario haircut. This one was far enough away that we had to hop in our car to get to it, but once we were there, it offered up a beautiful walking trail, a full-mile loop around even more unexpected beauty right there in the middle of our city. Emma Prusch Farm Park was an old working farm that had been donated to the City of San Jose. It had an old barn, which the city converted into an educational center, and an old-fashioned windmill that squeaked a bit as it turned in the breeze. While the sound of cars on the nearby freeway filtered through the air like distant ocean waves, the lawns and bushes produced a different sound that immediately caught Peety's attention: the sound of chickens. The "cluck, cluck, cluck" of those birds, and the occasional call of a rooster, made it feel like we'd traveled far out into the countryside. And while Peety wasn't allowed off leash in this park—there were too many people sunbathing or walking with their own dogs for me to even think about it—it instantly became one of his favorite places to go. Yes, he tugged on the end of the leash and tried to run after the chickens. Yes, he yanked me forward as he barked at other dogs. But he loved the sights and smells and excitement around every corner.

So did I.

For some reason, this particular park was a hotspot for women and their dogs to exercise, and for the first time in years, I found myself noticing those women. Fifteen years is a long time to go without a date, and clearly the supplements Dr. Preeti had given me (combined with my change in lifestyle) were beginning to kick in, because every time we walked around that park, I found myself checking someone out. The sensations caught me off guard. A whiff of perfume. A long blond ponytail bouncing in time with a jog. Bare shoulders in a tank top.

A lot had changed in terms of workout fashion in the fifteen years since I'd taken myself off the market. Women now wore yoga pants, which are pretty much just tights. In public. With nothing over them. I was almost embarrassed to look sometimes! But the shocking part is that I found myself looking at all.

Peety drew all sorts of attention from women of all ages at the Farm. "What a cutey!" "Well, hi there! Aren't you adorable." Peety loved it. He absolutely preened whenever someone rubbed his neck. Yet these women didn't look at me with the same affection. I was still huge. Even as I dropped below three hundred pounds, and stuck to my animal-free diet, and found myself taking longer and longer walks with Peety on the weekends, there was nothing attractive about me other than my dog. I was positive that if I'd walked through that park alone, not one of those women would have looked me in the eye, let alone stopped to say hello to me. Even with my handsome new Mario-given haircut.

Still, the fact that I felt even moderately attracted to some of those women gave me hope. Maybe if I continued to get healthier, someday one of those women might look in my direction, and actually be attracted—to *me*.

Beyond my sudden awareness of the bevy of blondes and brunettes at that park, though, I discovered the existence of something I had never paid attention to in my life: a farmer's market. Once a week, a whole bunch of farmers from the surrounding area would set up tents and tables and hock their fresh-from-the-farm fruits and vegetables in that park. I had never seen such amazing-looking food in my life. I lived in California, the land of plenty, where fresh produce is grown year-round. Yet I hadn't bought fresh produce in years, and I had never purchased it directly from those who grew it. I can't even imagine what some of those farmers must have thought of me as I marveled at their products.

Peety strutted through the market on patrol, sniffing and evaluating as we went along. "What do you think, Peety?" I'd ask him, holding a tomato or zucchini down to let him sniff. He'd look up at me to approve, or look away to deny. The vendors, most of whom were Mexican, didn't seem to mind at all that a dog was examining their produce. They were very accepting of Peety's presence, and more than a few of them offered him treats along the way. Some even had home-baked dog treats available for purchase. Having a dog at a farmer's market seemed just as organic as the new fruits and vegetables I discovered at every turn.

I, on the other hand, felt like an alien dropped here from another planet, completely amazed and bewildered by everything I saw. There were heirloom tomatoes in all sorts of odd shapes, sizes, and colors. I never knew a tomato could be anything but red and round! There were yellow ones, and purple ones, and some that were almost black, and some near white. A whole rainbow could be found in just the tomato bins. I picked up a zucchini that was bigger than the largest extra-large steak-and-cheese sub I'd ever consumed. There were oranges of all different sizes, and nectarines, and apricots, and all sorts of fresh lettuces and greens, and almonds, and avocados ripe and ready for eating, and cantaloupes that smelled delicious right through their skin.

The farm park also offered a farm-share or CSA (Community Supported Agriculture) option, where a person could pay a few hundred dollars to pre-purchase a six-month supply of fruits and vegetables. Then every week, the farms would load up a box full of food just for you, filled to the brim with whatever fruits and veggies were ripe and ready that particular week. You would never know exactly what you were going to get. You'd just come and pick up your box—and to me, in the middle of my adventure of discovering new foods, that only added to the appeal.

I signed up on the spot. I ran the numbers in my head, and the sheer volume of food I would receive through that farm-share system meant I would be saving a ton of money on groceries. I could hardly believe it: hand-grown, just-cut produce was going to make its way directly from the earth to my kitchen for what amounted to pennies on the dollar.

In fact, this entire diet was turning into a money-saving

bonanza. I found I could buy organic tofu for $1.20 a pound at Costco. For $12, I could buy massive bags of beans or rice that would last months and cost just pennies per serving. I invested in some good food-storage bins so everything would stay fresh and organized in the pantry, and I found I could feed myself for less than half as much as any average meat-based meals would cost—even when I started to buy as much fresh, local, organic product as possible. Compared to my old ways of delivery and window dining, I found myself eating for what was often less than a quarter of the cost per meal.

Plus, it was just plain fun. I followed Dr. Preeti's advice and started shopping at Mexican and Asian markets instead of my standard American supermarkets, and every time I walked through those doors I discovered foods that I had never seen before. Or smelled before. There were whole aisles dedicated to nothing but dried spices. Not little jars of ground-up spices, but bags and bins full of whole chilies and leaves, seeds, stems, and roots of plants that had been dried and were ready for fresh grinding in the kitchen, which made the flavors ten times more potent and pungent and wonderful than anything that came out of a jar. There seemed to be new vegetables on display every trip I made, too. One week I discovered bok choy, a nutrient-dense rich green leafy vegetable that stir-fried into the most amazing texture and flavor with nothing but a little garlic and a few flakes of red pepper. Another week, I walked by cases of jackfruit at the entryway, these incredible-looking, oddly shaped, gigantic green orbs that were larger than a human head. I didn't dare take one home. They looked like something that must have grown on monstrous trees in the age of dinosaurs. But I read about them and discovered that more and more top vegan chefs were using the jackfruit's meaty texture in cooking, sometimes to replicate the look and feel of pulled pork on their menus.

The richness of all of the sights and smells and smiles of the patrons in those stores that I'd driven right by in the past made me want to return again and again. I couldn't get enough. I kept thinking about Dr. Preeti's revelation that there were more than twenty thousand edible plants in the world, and I wanted to try them all!

And that fascination fed my hunger to want to learn all I could about how to prepare these brand-new foods that kept finding their way into my kitchen.

Of course, around all of this blissful new earthly discovery, Peety and I had to deal with real life, too. And life always has a way of throwing stuff at you when you least expect it. Especially little annoying things, like when you get up to flush one random Sunday morning and the handle falls off your toilet.

That was definitely not how I wanted to start my day. I lifted up the cover on the back of the commode and was able to pull the rod to flush it by hand, but I quickly realized that the handle didn't just come loose. It actually broke. It was a cheaply made toilet. And since this wasn't a rental apartment, I didn't have a super to call to come fix it. That meant I needed to either hire a plumber or fix it myself.

Since I knew no plumber would show up on a Sunday without charging a jacked-up "emergency rate," I told Peety

I'd be back and I headed off to the Home Depot with the broken handle in my hand.

The old me would have been in and out of that store as fast as possible. I would have looked online first, at a map of the store, so I could find the shortest route to the plumbing section and back. Actually, now that I think about it, the old me might have left the top off of the toilet and just continued to flush it by pulling the rod. Forever. But I certainly wouldn't have stopped and lingered in the lighting section as I walked to the back of the Home Depot. I would never have let my eye wander long enough to think about what one of the more wild-looking modern chandeliers with bright red blown-glass shades might look like in my dining area. I certainly wouldn't have wandered over to poke around the shelving and storage units, with thoughts of organizing my work files so I could clear off that dining room table. I never would have wandered into the paint section, or the power tools section, or the blinds and drapery section, just to poke around and see how much things cost. Once I finally trekked all the way back to the front of the store, near the registers, I never would have stopped to look at the decorating books, or to pick up a woodworking book on easy projects to complete for your home. But I did. I did *all* of those things. I spent the better part of my Sunday wandering around the Home Depot.

I had been pretty handy as a kid. I was a standout student in shop class and woodworking class. But I hadn't picked up a hammer and a nail to do anything other than hang a picture in years, and I hadn't even done *that* since I moved into my condo a year before Peety came into my life. So it was almost an out-of-body experience to watch the checkout girl ring up the toilet tank repair kit, and the woodworking book, and two decorating books.

*I'm really gonna do this*, I thought.

Then I *did*.

I read those books cover to cover, gathering ideas and making plans in my head. I learned about color wheels, and hues, and that the main thing I needed in order to achieve decorating success was to build around a particular theme, or color, or object. I found myself so enamored with the Mexican heritage of my newly discovered neighborhood that I decided to use that as my design. The warmth of Spanish architecture and the boldness of Mexican-style color palettes felt rich and inviting to me now—and the white walls of my apartment felt more bare and empty than ever.

So I trekked out to Kelly-Moore and picked up two giant buckets of paint in a color named Cream Cake. That's where I would start: getting rid of the white walls. Peety followed me from room to room and watched with amazement as I painted every wall in that condo. Then he did it again as I returned from the paint store with a whole host of colors from the store's Spanish Revival palette, and started painting different-colored bold accent walls of chocolate brown and terra cotta and more, with a different colored wall in every room. I bought work lights so I could continue painting at night, and when I wasn't walking with Peety on the weekends, I dedicated most of my free hours to transforming my apartment into something we could truly be proud of.

Instead of buying the chandeliers I saw at Home Depot, I went to lighting centers and found super high-end fixtures that were slightly damaged or had just been returned, so I could purchase the highest quality products possible at a deep discount. I decided to get rid of the twenty-cent plastic switch plates on all of my light switches and electrical outlets, too, replacing them with beautiful, handmade painted steel and glass switch plates in all sorts of colors to match my theme. That one tiny detail made such a huge difference in every room. For an investment of a couple hundred dollars, it made the difference between staying at a Super 8 Motel and vacationing at a beautiful five-star resort.

I installed a custom, stainless-steel, overhead pot rack above the island in the kitchen and displayed my whole array of new restaurant-quality pots and pans like something you'd see in a gourmet restaurant. I taught myself how to work with tile and grout and installed an exotic glass backsplash in my kitchen, too.

Then I went back to Home Depot and picked up some power tools and quickly got about making handcrafted window cornices, end tables, and good-looking step stools, shelves, and plant stands to keep around the house. I designed them with details that matched what I saw in picture books of Spanish architecture, then stained them in a deep rich brown. My neighbors probably hated me for all the noise I made doing that woodworking, but I couldn't stop myself. Once I got going, once I saw that I could put my personal touch on this space, and have it come out looking good, I kept wanting to do more. I enjoyed the smell of the sawdust. Peety would come over and roll in it like he was taking a scratchy bath, and I'd brush it off of him with a towel before vacuuming it all up. The noise didn't bother him one bit. And when we got hungry, the two of us ate our meals together, sitting on the living room floor.

Sitting on that floor night after night got me thinking about all sorts of things, just like it had on the night of our first shared tofu stir-fry. First and foremost, I decided that the laminate flooring we were sitting on was just too run-of-the-mill. Peety deserved something a whole lot better. So I bought, laid out, cut, and installed a Brazilian-cherry hardwood floor. That meant getting down on the ground, in kneepads, and tapping and gluing that flooring into place. It was backbreaking work. *Knee*-breaking work. I had to spread it out over several days, working in small intervals so I wouldn't hurt myself. I got winded while I worked. I got sweaty. But Peety kept licking the saltiness from my cheeks, and his looks of admiration kept me going.

Working around my work schedule and my long weekend walks with Peety, it took me a couple of months to get the stage set. But soon enough, the walls, the floors, the lighting—all the basics were complete. Peety and I no longer found ourselves living in a plain white box. Every single time we opened the door and turned on the lights we felt a sense of surprise and a jolt of pride. The warm colors and textures of our home made us both feel like we were stepping into something much more than a condo. Together, we were stepping into our palace.

The best part was I knew it wasn't finished. This was a work in progress. The cheap prints I finally took out of boxes and hung on the walls didn't match the quality of my handiwork. By comparison, they looked like leftovers from somebody's college dorm room. I had poured my heart into making this place look good, and I decided that needed to continue. I needed a real bed frame. With a headboard. Maybe even a footboard. I'd never owned a bed like that. The Ikea dresser seemed wholly insufficient. The dining room table was nothing special. Now that I had shelves up, and the boxes were gone, and there was a beautiful chandelier overhead, and now that I was cooking all of this fantastic food, didn't we deserve a dining room table befitting all of that?

I can't fully explain why the feeling came over me that I wanted to fill our home with nothing but beautiful things. It just did. And I can't explain why ordering furnishings online and having them delivered from some anonymous warehouse somewhere completely lost its appeal. But it did. I had transformed our home with my own two hands. And from that point forward, I felt as if everything that came into that home ought to have been loved and cared for in the same manner.

And that made me think: perhaps Peety and I needed to make it our mission to go find things like that, wherever they may be. And the first thing we needed was some art.

"Peety," I said. "How would you like to take our next big walk in San Francisco?"

# chapter 10

## Progress

In the first three months, every time I visited Dr. Preeti's office to get on the scale, I took off my shoes, and my belt, and I made sure to wear the lightest clothing I owned. I even cut back on salt in the hopes that I'd shed some water weight before walking in to our weekly meeting. I did it all because I wanted to impress her, to make sure she saw how great I was doing. It took me a little while to realize that the pounds I lost from week to week didn't actually matter to her. I suppose if I started gaining weight she might have expressed some concern, but that's all it would have been. Not shame. Not a scolding. Concern. She was my champion. She wanted me to succeed. This wasn't a race. This wasn't a competition. This wasn't school. I wouldn't be graded on my performance. All she cared about is that I was feeling better. When she did talk numbers, it was more about inches and percentage of body fat than "weight." All she wanted was for me to get healthy. And I *was*.

I also reached a point where I no longer felt like I had

to work at this diet plan. The work of it just sort of faded into the background. I ate plant-based foods. That's what I ate. Nothing else. I took walks twice a day with Peety. I took longer walks with him on the weekends. I did my work. I tried new recipes now and then. I kept my housecleaner on, even though Peety wasn't nearly as messy as he'd been in the beginning, and I hired her to come by and walk him when I had to go out of town on business, because I couldn't stand the thought of putting Peety into a kennel. My home was his home and he deserved to stay in his home. I desperately wished I could have found some way to bring him with me on trips, and to business meetings, and just about everywhere, but I was pretty sure the business world wouldn't accept the presence of a fifty-pound dog. So I made all of my trips as short as possible, and I cut down on them as much as I possibly could.

As the months went by, these things just became my routine. They were my life. Losing weight just seemed to be a by-product of it all rather than the primary motivation.

In fact, the way I lived with Peety had become such a routine, I didn't even realize I'd reached my six-month anniversary with Dr. Preeti. I was shocked when I walked into her office and she told me this was my last pre-paid weekly visit. We would be cutting back to once a month follow-up appointments, she said, if I was comfortable with that.

I was sad about it. I kind of liked coming in and telling her about everything I'd been eating, and where I'd gone, and how great Peety was doing, and how much better I felt. But of course, I also marked it as a major milestone: Dr. Preeti felt I was ready to do this on my own now. The monthly check-ins were important, she said, until I reached a fully healthy weight and she was able to take me off the rest of the supplements, and my blood work was normal. But my blood work was *already* remarkably normal.

In less than six months, I'd managed to stop taking every medication I was on. I was off insulin, with normal glucose and A1C levels. My total cholesterol had dropped from almost 400 to 120, and my blood pressure was down from 170/100 to 100/60. With every medication Dr. Preeti weaned me off of, I found myself feeling even better than I'd felt before. I swear half of my problems, including some of my joint pain, some of the upset stomach and bowel symptoms, the sleep issues, the fatigue, the headaches, and more, were nothing but side effects from the medications I was taking to try to keep me alive in my morbidly obese state. I'd turned into a living, breathing, barely walking human billboard promoting the long list of awful side effects the pharmaceutical companies warn us about in TV commercials for new drugs.

I was still overweight. I still had a long way to go by any normal standards. But at my six-month check-in with Dr. Preeti, as I stood barefoot on that doctor's scale with its cold black metal base and the white stem leading up to the portion with the sliders on top that move side to side to determine your fate, I watched as she pushed the slider down, down, down, farther to the left than it had ever been pushed in my presence—all the way down to 210 pounds.

In just six months, by simply following this doctor's orders—which, when it came right down to it, meant eating a bunch of really delicious food, and taking walks with my dog, who I loved, and who loved me back—I had dropped the weight of a healthy, full-grown, five-foot-four adult woman. I'd been carrying around the weight of an adult human being! I Googled it and found that 120 pounds is the equivalent of carrying ten gallons of full paint cans around your waist; or 150 cans of soup. Some appliances I sold weighed less than the amount of weight I'd dropped in the course of those twenty-four weeks.

I thought about every other diet plan I'd ever tried, and I felt like such a fool. I felt like I'd been duped. *Why did no one tell me about this plant-based solution before? Why isn't this plan Dr. Preeti put me on the sensation that the whole dieting world is talking about? Why don't doctors tell us how effective this diet change can be? How is it that average people don't know how effective this is, and how simple this is?*

I tried not to focus on the number. The weight loss was just a side effect of eating healthy and light exercise. I knew that. Still: *A hundred and twenty pounds?*

I could feel my eyes welling up with tears as I stood there.

"Thank you," I said.

"Well, thank you for being such a good patient, Eric," Dr. Preeti said. "You really should thank yourself. You're the one who made the choice and commitment to come this far."

"But I couldn't have come this far without you," I said.

"I'm just happy to see you feeling better. And I hope you continue."

"Oh, I will. No doubt. I will never, ever, ever go back to the way things were," I said.

"Just remember, it's what you do on a daily basis that matters. I love to hear that you're taking long walks on the weekends, but keep up the thirty minutes twice a day, every day. That's the key. Be consistent, and don't try to make up for lost time by missing days and trying to double or triple up later."

"OK," I said.

"And when I don't see you every week, try to keep up as if you were coming here to check in. You might want to keep a scale at home if you find that a motivating factor. Keep eating well, of course. If you're getting bored with your meals, be sure to try something new. There's always something new without having to slip back to eating ani—"

"Oh, I'm not going back. I promise. I don't even want to. I smell a hamburger now and it doesn't even smell good to me," I told her. "The thought of eating animal flesh now seems gross to me. And in fact, I'm thinking about trying to find some plant-based cooking classes or something. I never want to get bored with my food choices, you know? I want to keep learning. I want to learn to cook really well, to cook new meals for Peety, too. He loves the food I make for him."

"Great! Go for it. Anything that keeps you engaged. And a cooking class could be a good social activity as well, if it's a group class. Sharing recipes with others, cooking together, sharing meals together—not just with Peety but with other people with similar tastes and interests—that could help you to stay focused and on track."

"Yeah," I said. "I hope you don't think it's too weird that I have dinner with my dog most nights."

"No! I'm not knocking that at all. But, you know, have you thought about trying to join any social groups, or to date again, or anything like that?"

"No. Not really. I mean…I'm not in any shape to catch someone's eye, you know. There's a long way to—"

"Don't count yourself out, Eric. Sometimes the way you see yourself doesn't match the way the rest of the world sees you. It may take you a long time to catch up and stop seeing yourself how you were, but you're not that same person in so many ways. Look at everything you've been up to, with your woodworking and remodeling…"

I wasn't buying it. I wasn't ready to date. I was sure no woman would be interested in me. But I had reasons besides my weight to stay away from dating, too. There was something going on with my body that didn't make any sense to me, and I found it grotesque and embarrassing. I thought I'd have to deal with folds of extra skin after losing weight so quickly, but that wasn't the case. I guess I was lucky in that regard, the way some women have the genetics to bounce right back into shape after pregnancy with hardly a stretch mark. My skin seemed to shrink back to normal in relative proportion to the pounds I lost. So it wasn't that. It was something else.

I wasn't ready to share it—not even with Dr. Preeti. It would take me another couple of months, and making the mistake of seeing another doctor to try to take care of the problem, before I would finally talk with her about it. But I knew that until it went away, there was no chance I could ever get close to a woman.

Still, I appreciated what Dr. Preeti was saying. Once again, it gave me hope that I was getting closer to the possibility of leading some sort of a normal life.

When I left her office that afternoon, I did so with less of a feeling of triumph than one of wondering when it would end. The self-doubt. The misery. The way every time things seemed to be going well, something new and terrible would always crop up.

I tried to find solace in my memories of Scripture. I still kept the Bible next to my bed. I opened it up every now and then, just to remind myself of the power of those words. I recalled a Psalm:

> *Wait patiently for the Lord.*
> *Be brave and courageous.*
> *Yes, wait patiently for the Lord.*
> —Psalm 27:14 (NLT)

I broke down and cried in my car in the parking lot. Here I was, 120 pounds lighter and feeling like my body was betraying me.

Underneath my clothes, my plaque psoriasis had grown exponentially worse. It had spread. It was itchy. It was painful. The scaly look of it made me feel like some sort of reptile. And the place where it was showing up seemed downright cruel—as if I were being punished by God Himself.

The grotesque betrayal of my own skin made me doubt myself. I doubted my ability to carry on. I doubted whether any of this had been worth it. I thought about Peety, and I shook my head, and I took a deep breath. I knew I couldn't leave him. I couldn't check out. It wasn't so bad that I was thinking about suicide. Those sorts of thoughts hadn't entered my head since I'd seen the light. But I didn't know how to escape the awful feeling that something was terribly, terribly wrong with me.

I wanted to be patient. I knew I needed to carry on. To keep going. I was excited to take Peety to San Francisco that weekend. I was excited to take him all over the place. I just wished I could take him everywhere with me.

When I was apart from him, I missed him. And that's when I found myself falling back into the space I'd been in before. Alone. Isolated. Lonely. Disconnected from the world.

On the few short business trips I'd taken since bringing Peety home, I'd spent every hour that I wasn't working locked in my hotel room. I ordered room service, knowing there wasn't a single option for me to eat besides salads and potatoes. And it was so much effort sometimes explaining to kitchen staff what "vegan" meant. It meant, "Do not cook my potatoes in butter or add butter, sour cream, or cheese to anything." Even after all of that I would sometimes have to send my food back. They would sprinkle cheese all over my salad, along with croutons and dressing that were likely made with dairy and eggs and were certainly steeped in all sorts of artificial ingredients.

If I could have brought Peety along on those trips, I knew his presence would have made everything so much easier. Nothing seemed to get me down as long as I could look in Peety's eyes.

I had so much to be thankful for. I was genuinely happy on so many days now. And yet, even that happiness seemed to be missing something. More than ever, and truly for the first time in two decades, I genuinely wished that I had another person to share things with. No one but Peety and my housekeeper Sally had seen any of the work I'd done in my condo. Sure, I had shown Dr. Preeti some cell phone pics of my shelves and my cool new paint job, but that was it. Except for the smiles and hellos from my new friends in Mario's neighborhood, I didn't share a whole lot of interaction with any other human beings. Especially when Peety wasn't with me.

"God," I prayed, "please allow me to have a normal life."

I drove home that afternoon ticking off the years in my head, trying to remember the last time I felt "normal."

*Man, oh, man,* I thought. *It's been a really, really long time since the gloriousness of normalcy was anything I knew.*

# chapter 11

# Pudgeville

Pudge! Pudge!! Get the ball! Go get it!!"

Tim was the most athletic kid of them all. I was out in
center field. It was third grade. We were playing a game of
gym-class kickball, and Tim had kicked that red rubber ball
all the way over my head and straight over the chain-link
fence.

Suddenly all the rest of the kids joined in his cry. "Go get
it, Pudge!" "Come on, Pudge!"

I turned and walked back to the fence as fast as I could
while Tim rounded the bases. It wasn't a tall fence. It was
only as tall as me, just a perimeter marker around the field.
But to me, it might as well have been the Great Wall of
China. I grabbed the top bar and put one foot up, trying to
wedge my shoe into the diamond-shaped hole, but the grass
was covered in dew. My shoe slipped out as soon as I put
any weight on it. I tried to hold the top bar and throw my leg
up over it so I could hoist myself over the fence, but my leg
wouldn't reach that high.

"Come on, Pudge!" they yelled.

I could feel my face burning red as I put both hands in the top bar and jumped, trying to somehow lift myself straight up on both arms like an Olympian on the high bar. I held myself there for a good three seconds, my feet flailing, trying to grab a toehold to give me the extra push. I didn't care if I flipped right over and fell on the other side. I needed to get over that fence!

But I couldn't.

In the time I spent trying, Tim rounded the bases, touched home plate to win the game, and ran all the way out into center field. Without stopping, without hesitation, he came flying toward the fence, threw one arm forward, and catapulted himself right over it. He landed on his feet on the other side, picked up the ball, and threw it so hard it bounced all the way into the arms of our gym teacher at the pitcher's mound.

I'm not sure why I thought of that moment right then. It wasn't a pivotal moment for me or anything like that. I didn't break down in tears on that day. The kids didn't taunt me relentlessly. It was just another day in third grade, like any other day when I found myself unable to do what others could do simply because I was overweight.

My gym teacher didn't scold anyone for calling me Pudge, because everyone called me Pudge. It was just a nickname. *Like anyone else's nickname*, I thought.

Pudge was who I was.

My parents divorced when I was twelve, and my mom moved out. My dad worked three jobs and was always gone. He would drop by at least once a week to fill up the refrigerator and the cupboards with groceries, and then he'd leave again. I'm sure he was there more often than that, but none of us would have known it. After the divorce, he became sort of a ladies' man. He was always with someone new. And in the absence of adult supervision, the seven of us kids—my two brothers and the four siblings my parents had adopted when my mom's sister passed away—basically turned into hoodlums. I won't get into the finer details of what went on, but trouble seemed to follow us around. This was the San Francisco Bay Area in the 1960s and early 1970s. Pot smoking was a given for just about every kid I knew. In fact, I had started smoking cigarettes and weed by age thirteen. But with us, it went a whole lot further than normal teenage rebellion. I saw money, and guns, and let's just say that our crew may have stolen a car on more than one occasion.

The only peace I found was in the arms of my girlfriend. Jaye was a year younger than me, and easily the most accepting, loving person I had ever met. The two of us cut school sometimes just so we could spend the day together. I'd grown a few inches by junior year, and I wasn't quite as pudgy as I'd been in my Pudge past, but I was certainly no looker when compared to most of my peers.

Jaye didn't care about that. She looked at me like I was the most attractive guy she'd ever seen. She loved me simply for being me. And I loved her right back.

We dated for two years. Heck, we might have gotten married if fate hadn't pushed us apart.

By the time I was seventeen, my friends got mixed up in some really bad stuff. I saw the road they were on and knew I needed to choose a different path. If I didn't get out of there, I feared I was going to wind up dead or in prison. So I joined the army. I escaped about as far from home as I could get. I wound up stationed in Germany, and I hated every minute of it. Jaye and I lost touch, while the army whipped my body into shape through force. I got "fit" because the food was terrible and I hated eating it, and because the army forced me to endure strenuous daily physical training.

I hate to break it to you, but that isn't "fit" at all. It's torture.

When I finally got out of the army, I hitchhiked and drifted around the country, ending up in Kansas. I found a job painting water towers for $13 an hour. This was the early '80s, so $13 an hour was a lot of money. But the work was hard and dangerous. I'd be over a hundred feet in the air on these towers, working inside of a steel tank in 120-degree heat, sandblasting and painting with epoxy-based paint. The fumes were often so bad and the oxygen system so poor that I'd wind up hallucinating.

The job didn't last, but it did teach me one great life lesson: I knew I never wanted to do physical labor again if I could avoid it.

I went back to the Bay Area and realized that I had no idea what I wanted to do with my life. I figured I needed to explore. So I went to a temp agency and said, "I want to work, but I want you to put me in a different job every week for an entire year. Never the same job twice. Never the same *field* twice if you can avoid it."

The temp agency came through. I worked fifty-two jobs in fifty-two weeks, and what I basically discovered is there are two types of jobs: there are jobs where you get paid to use your body, often in the heat of the sun, and there are jobs where you get paid to use your mind. Those jobs usually involve sitting inside a comfortable, air-conditioned building.

I decided to choose the life of the latter.

After some trial and error with different companies, I discovered that I was really good at sales. I could talk to people, and listen to people, and get along with people, and laugh with people, and basically help them understand that what I was asking them to do was simply in their best interest. My basic motivation in life became to make as much money as possible by doing the least amount of work possible. The sales themselves weren't really work. That was kind of fun. What I mean is the work of dealing with bosses, with all of the headaches and the micromanagement people throw at you in an attempt to control you and make you feel small. I hated being controlled. I got out of the army and never wanted to be told what to do again. I know that's not entirely possible in life, but I sure tried my best to make my life work out that way.

I finally figured out that the best sales job in the world was working as a salesman on the West Coast—for a manufacturing company headquartered somewhere back East. That way you'd have all the corporate backing and expense accounts you'd need to get the job done while living on your own time clock, basically making your own schedule with only occasional visits from bosses or managers, and the *very* occasional trip to some remote headquarters. The consumer goods industry seemed to offer the best opportunities in that area, and so that's what I pursued.

I made good money, and my army-abused body lasted me

well into my late twenties. I was a good-looking young guy with money to burn, and my dating life was on fire. I had fun. But that bouncing around from person to person gets old pretty quick. And with the traveling I had to do for the company I worked for at that time, I was never in one place for very long.

I found myself thinking about wanting a more stable life. Maybe a wife. But I also wanted a good life. One where I didn't have to worry about money all the time like my parents did. I wasn't sure how to get both of those.

At parties and bars, I always found myself dodging certain questions, too, like, "Where'd you go to college?" There were times when I felt like I was the only guy in California without a college degree. The women I was attracted to always seemed turned off that I hadn't gone to school. I felt like my lack of a degree was holding me back in my career, and in my life. *What kind of a woman would want to marry an uneducated guy like me?*

I didn't know anything about getting into college. I had no idea how to apply, or if an older guy like me could even get into a school this late in life. So I used my salesman skills and made some cold calls. I wound up getting an appointment with the president of San Jose State University, and he told me about College Level Examination Program tests I could take that would allow me to meet most of my first-year class requirements by testing, rather than by taking bonehead English and math classes. If I passed those exams, he said, I'd be admitted.

That was all I needed to know.

I studied my butt off. I read and read. I purchased and

worked my way through books such as *Teach Yourself Long Division and Fractions*. I ended up teaching myself all of the math I never bothered to learn in high school, and when I took my tests, I passed them all. I tested out of my entire freshman year of required course work. For the next three years, while still holding down a sales job, I worked my tail off and completed my bachelor's degree in high style: I graduated summa cum laude at the head of my class.

At that point, I had options. I decided that the guys who really made all the money in life, win or lose, no matter what the economy was, were lawyers. And what were lawyers but great salespeople who convinced judges and juries to buy what they were selling? It was a perfect match.

I applied to law school and was accepted by my top-two choices: Stanford and Emory. I should have gone to Stanford. It would have led me down a different path, I think. But Emory University offered me a full scholarship—basically an all-expense-paid fellowship through school, including tuition, books, and living expenses, absolutely everything I would need to get through law school and succeed. It was a gift too good to pass up. So I packed my things and headed to Atlanta.

In law school, I stopped exercising and wasn't playing any sports or getting any kind of physical activity, which marked the start of my return to Pudgeville. I ballooned up quickly, thanks in part to the seemingly never-ending supply of barbecue, fried chicken, and biscuits with white gravy in Atlanta.

By the time I passed the bar exam, I was more than just heavyset. I was on my way to obesity.

After landing a plum first-year-associate position at the Atlanta office of one of the world's largest law firms, I found myself hating always answering to the man. I hated the micromanagement. I hated having to constantly check in with bosses to prove myself while working twelve hours a day or longer for the chance to climb the law firm ladder. I wasn't in my twenties. I didn't feel like grinding for eight or ten years in the hopes of making partner. So I decided to strike out on my own. I opened my own one-man law firm and made a niche for myself defending drug dealers. I figured there was a never-ending supply of customers, and I knew more than a little something about that world from hanging out with my crew back in high school.

I left my business cards in every phone booth in every bad neighborhood in Atlanta. I made sure my clients wrote my phone number next to the pay phone inside every jail before they bailed out. Before long, I was the go-to guy for every major drug dealer in metro Atlanta. I was making money hand over fist. I drove a big purple Chevy convertible with shiny rims so I'd never go unnoticed, and I'd drive up to the window at Popeyes to order big buckets of fried chicken to eat while I drove around to visit my clients in jail.

The only problem was I started to feel sick. My weight soon ballooned up to two hundred fifty pounds. My knees started to hurt so much I'd have to sit down even when I should have been standing in the courtroom. I had money, and health insurance, so I went to see doctors to see if they could help me. They told me to go on a diet. They told me to exercise. Then they handed me a prescription instead. It started with Adderall, but the results were minimal. I was so desperate to lose weight and to stop feeling miserable that I went back to the doctor and asked for a stronger prescription. They moved up to Ritalin, then Dexedrine, then Desoxyn, which is the legal prescription form of methamphetamine.

Even then, they would never give me enough to take all the weight off.

My clients were all drug dealers.

You can see where this is going.

One day, talking about my weight dilemma with a client, she offered to give me some of her product. The methamphetamine she provided worked exactly as the prescription form did, but my supply wasn't limited. So I took as much as I wanted. I began losing the weight I wanted to shed. I also enjoyed the elation of getting high and forgetting about all of my troubles and pain. Soon, the weight loss became a secondary motive. Before long, I wanted—and needed—to keep that high.

The thing you learn when you represent drug dealers is that the police and the DEA and the prosecutors have quite a racket going. They build their cases on the backs of drug dealers ratting each other out. They can go to a magistrate with sketchy information to establish probable cause and obtain search warrants fairly easily. And if they don't want to bother getting a legal warrant, they can concoct scenarios to stop and frisk almost anyone they choose. It's an ugly business that's perpetuated by a broken system—and I hated that system. While high as a kite, I started giving seminars to drug users. I taught them never to talk to cops. I taught them their rights. I gave them stacks of cards to carry with them at all times, so if they ever got pulled over they could hand the officer my card and immediately invoke their right to an attorney without saying a single word. I decided to buck the system, to rebuke "the man," and to help give the little people some power for once.

Needless to say, this didn't make the local law enforcement community happy.

I quickly became a target.

They flipped one of my clients in a plea bargain, and she gave me up. She gave me up just so she could avoid booking and bail.

I walked out of court one day to find my purple convertible surrounded by cops. I knew it was over. I had a small, personal-use quantity of speed in my pocket, and the officers discovered it while patting me down for weapons.

I wound up making a deal for myself. I took the punishment that would keep me out of jail while still keeping my integrity. I surrendered my law license and accepted a first-offender plea under Georgia law, which meant that once I completed my probation, all of my civil rights would be restored and I could, by law, state that I had never been convicted of the crime. I could have stuck around and eventually reapplied for my law license if I wanted to. But I didn't want to. I sold everything I owned, including my purple Chevy. I bought a bus ticket to San Francisco and I went home, to start my life over.

I spent the next year broke, unemployed, and lamenting my situation. I sent out more than five hundred résumés and got no interest from anyone. I figured nobody wanted to hire a disbarred attorney on probation, and it was all too difficult to explain. Which pretty much meant that I had to leave the whole five-year-long "attorney" part of my job history off of my résumé. That left me whittling away at what little money I had in the bank until there was nothing left. It's quite a shock going from making serious money to being flat broke. Finally, when I ran out of food and was about to get evicted from my room at a pay-by-the-week hotel, I decided to fall back into the only field I knew: sales. I knew I wouldn't be able to start at the top, so I flipped a coin between taking a job at Home Depot or Fry's Electronics. Fry's won the toss. I went in, head hung low, and in two months I worked my way up from sales associate, to department manager, to appliance buyer for thirty-four stores. After two years as a buyer for Fry's, I landed a job in field sales with a major appliance manufacturer.

Without weight-loss drugs and with no desire to get hooked on any drug ever again, my weight ballooned up twice as fast as it had in Georgia. My metabolism bottomed out once I hit my early forties. I lost my ability to shop at Nordstrom. I soared to over three hundred pounds. It hurt just to walk. It hurt to fly. It hurt just to lie down in bed.

I moved into my new white box of a condo in East San Jose and closed the door.

Like I said, it had been a very long time since I'd enjoyed anything close to that thing most people call "normal."

# chapter 12

# The Bridge

I'd spent six months making all sorts of new discoveries, but then I fell into a rut. When it came to food, I had hit a wall.

I found myself making the same dishes over and over again, just because they were easy. Especially pasta. Not wheat-based pasta, but rice-based pasta. My favorite brand, Tinkyada, tasted exactly like regular pasta, but without gluten and with all the nutrition of brown rice. I made my own tomato sauce so I could be sure of every ingredient that went into it, buying fresh tomatoes in season, or jarred tomatoes to avoid the BPAs in many canned tomatoes. The more I read about our food system, the more awful every prepackaged thing seemed to me. It just astounded me how many foods in this country included chemicals and other ingredients that were suspected carcinogens. Why would I want to consume any of that, even in tiny quantities, after putting in all of this effort to get healthy?

I made a great sauce. I made a variety of different sauces. But it all started to feel a bit too routine.

I also found it difficult to incorporate some vegetables into my diet. When I was a kid, we rarely ate vegetables, and when we did they usually came from cans. They were mushy, metallic tasting, and packed with a shelf life of years. The memory of those smells and tastes were hard to shake. In fact, vegetables were sometimes given to me as a punishment. So certain vegetables, from a very young age, triggered my gag reflex. When I smelled them or when I tried to eat them, I actually felt like vomiting.

Brussels sprouts were a big one. I can't eat them to this day. I never liked artichokes. I wasn't a cauliflower fan. I really didn't get eggplant—it was slimy, and I just didn't understand why anyone would want to eat it. Those aversions made it difficult to incorporate some of the new and similar vegetables I'd come across into my cooking. So I needed a fresh start. I wanted to learn how to take anything I picked up in my farm-share box or anywhere else and turn it into something wholly nutritious and delicious. I had reached my capacity as a cook, and I needed lessons.

I decided to take Peety along with me on sales calls that Friday. I was heading up to Berkeley, the home of the famously liberal college campus, the hippie capital of the world, and an area that had become a vegan mecca. I figured I could ask around there and come up with somebody who might teach me a thing or two about vegan cooking. There were restaurants and cafés all over that town with multiple vegetarian and vegan options on their menus, and even restaurants that were 100 percent vegan. Peety and I skipped breakfast at home just so we could eat out at one of those cool places.

I stopped into one of my stores before we looked for food, and I brought Peety right in with me. I'd mentioned him to the staff plenty of times before, so everyone was happy to see him. They all came around from behind the counter to meet him and pet him. They had just opened the doors, so there were no customers in the place yet. I figured nobody would mind, and I was right.

Peety walked into this fifteen-thousand-square-foot showroom full of big metal boxes and machines, and guardedly sniffed around looking for another dog behind the rows of refrigerators and stoves. He seemed a little dismayed not to find anything. There aren't many places in the world that a dog would walk into that no other animal had been in the past. It had to be confusing to his nose and the rest of his senses.

It was so beautiful to see the smiles pop up on everyone's faces as they watched Peety sniff around. It changed the whole energy of the store in a matter of minutes. No matter how many times it happens, I don't think I will ever get tired of seeing the positive effect one dog can have on an otherwise cold and sterile environment.

As I was getting ready to leave, though, the manager asked me to come into his office in the back. It was unusual. He seemed sort of somber.

"Look, Eric, I just want to let you know how sorry I am. And if there's anything we can do here, you know, to make things easier or help out in some way, we'd like to help."

"What are you talking about?" I asked him.

"I just—I know you don't ever talk about it, but the guys here were talking, and someone mentioned why you'd been losing all the weight. I mean, I lost my mom to cancer just two years ago now. Watched her whither away to nothing before she died. So I know how tough it is to ask for help, but—"

"Dude," I said, "I don't have cancer." The poor guy turned white as a sheet. "Is that what people are saying about me? No, no, not at all, man."

"Well," he said. "Whatever it is, I—"

"I'm not sick, Bill. I'm healthier than I've ever been in my life. I'm just eating really healthy, and exercising."

"Seriously?" he said, his eyes wide with astonishment and embarrassment. "Aw man, that's really—that's good news."

"Yeah, it is!"

I laughed, and he broke into a laugh, too.

"Is that why everyone's been so quiet when I walk in here? I thought you guys heard something negative from another sales rep or were looking to drop our brand or something," I said.

"No! No. Not at all. I'm sorry. It was just a misunderstanding I guess. I don't know. You know how people talk. You just look so different. I mean, I don't think I've ever seen anyone lose weight so fast, you know what I mean? Except on TV, like on *The Biggest Loser* or something."

"Jeesh. Do I look sick to you guys?"

"No! That's the thing. We were saying how good you look! Ronny was saying, 'If only he had lost the weight for a reason that wasn't so sad, the guy would be rockin'!'"

I laughed at that, and so did he.

Silly Ronny, the biggest practical joker I knew, had struck again.

"Woof!" Peety barked.

"Shhh, shhh…it's OK, son," I said, petting Peety's head and scratching him behind the ears. "Well, I'm not sick. Not at all. Look, I'd better go get him some breakfast. Please tell the rest of the guys that I'm fine. I'm better than fine. I'm doing great, OK?"

"You got it, Eric. Sorry about the misunderstanding. I'm so glad you're OK!"

"Yeah, me, too!"

I decided to take Peety to a vegetarian café just up the street. It was a beautiful day, so we sat at an outdoor spot where I could tie him to my chair and try to keep him quiet under the table. He was fine with people, but he still barked and yanked on the leash whenever another dog came around. I tried to pick a table far from the sidewalk so he couldn't see, but he still got up and barked to let a couple of other dogs know that this was our table, and he was protecting me, so they'd better steer clear if they knew what was good for them. I had to calm him down more than once before I even ordered.

We wound up eating a meal that looked and tasted almost exactly like an egg scrambler—only the eggs were made entirely of tofu. I could hardly believe how delicious it was. I put Peety's plate right down on the ground, and he gobbled up his serving, too. I just had to ask the chef how he did it. The waitress was kind enough to send him out, and he explained it was just some diced onions and peppers, turmeric for color, some salt and pepper, and some smoked paprika and vegetable broth for flavor.

"Man, that's awesome. You don't give cooking classes, do you?"

"No, man. Too busy," he said.

"Know anyone who does?"

"Yeah, actually, you should look up Philip Gelb. Unbelievable chef. He does classes and throws awesome dinner parties at his studio where he serves meals and has musicians play while he cooks a meal right in front of you. Awesome, awesome guy."

"Gelb. All right. I'll look him up," I said. "Thanks."

Peety and I then headed over to Paco Collars, a workshop I'd heard about from a woman we'd met at the Farm Park in San Jose. Her dog wore a beautiful leather collar, and I asked her where she got it. Paco was the place, she said, so I figured we ought to check it out while we were in town.

Paco Collars was set up in a little stand-alone pink building with light blue trim. A big sign on the front announced, "Yes, a store just for dog collars."

There were all these hippie guys sitting around tables inside making handmade collars. That's all they did, all day long, and that's really all they sold. They were stunning pieces of art, really. Every one of them was unique. They weren't cheap, but I wanted Peety to have the best. A handmade, artfully designed collar seemed perfectly in line with our new fixed-up home and the whole lifestyle we wanted to lead. So Peety left that shop wearing a beautiful collar dotted with shiny metal studs and fine turquoise. He really looked handsome!

We stopped in to see a few other clients that day. I made some phone calls while I let Peety play in a little fenced-in dog park. He was much calmer off leash in that environment. He seemed to recognize that the fenced-in area was like his own Doggie Disneyworld. There, just like at Petco, he was off the clock and ready for fun.

Then, rather than sit in traffic on the way home just to drive all the way back into San Francisco the next day, I decided we ought to spend the night. We found a pet-friendly hotel, and I was shocked when they charged me a $50 fee just to let Peety stay in the room.

"It's just in case of damage and for the added cleanup," the desk clerk explained.

*What a racket*, I thought. *I've seen plenty of human beings capable of doing a lot more damage to a hotel room than one dog.*

That night, I looked up Chef Philip Gelb on my laptop and found him right away. He was kind of a legend, it seemed, but I was a little confused. Nowhere on his "Sound and Savor" food blog did it say anything about being a vegan chef. His short bio read, "Chef and musician running a catering and personal chef business in the San Francisco Bay Area. Anything from a dinner for 2 to a party of 200. We also produce our own twice-monthly series of dinner/concerts of world-renowned musicians and my cuisine in intimate locales in Oakland. Gourmet cuisine for all!"

Philip had some upcoming classes listed, and the menus looked to be vegetarian at the very least, but I wasn't sure. I didn't want to enroll in a class that would teach me how to cook with cheese or dairy or meat. It would have been a waste of time and money. So I shot him an e-mail just to confirm what kind of cooking he taught.

The next day, Peety and I made our way into San Francisco. I had briefly worked at Ghirardelli Square, on the waterfront, when I was a teenager, so I knew the area well. I thought it would be a great place for Peety and me to take a walk together. I wanted to show him the sea lions and let him experience all the sights and smells that the San Francisco waterfront had to offer. But we were also on a mission. I hoped that there was still an open market of sorts along the west end of the waterfront, close to the Golden Gate. Back in the day, there used to be local artists there every weekend, selling their work to tourists. My hope was that I'd find an affordable painting in a style that would suit our newly refurbished home.

Peety was in heaven. Every inch of that walk was filled with luscious smells that kept him bouncing back and forth from side to side at the end of the leash. He pulled me onward like a kid in a candy store.

"Peety. Peety," I said, squatting down and asking him to sit when we got out near the end of Pier 39. "Listen, boy," I said. Just then, a sea lion cried out from its wooden perch below. Peety cocked his head to the side and looked at me wide eyed. "That's a sea lion, son. Want to go see 'em?"

Peety stood up and pulled me right up to the rail. He stuck his head through and stared at those sea lions all piled up in the sun, and as soon as he saw one of them slide off into the water with a splash, he started barking. That got all of those sea lions upset, and they started barking right back at him!

"OK, son, let's go. Let's go," I said. A few tourists scowled at us, as if we'd done something wrong; as if Peety had less of a right to be there than anyone else. So what if he barked?

The sea lions barked all they wanted with no complaints. Why couldn't my dog bark, too? It sounded like healthy interspecies communication to me.

The whole thing made me laugh. Back when I was a kid I never could have imagined I'd come back to this spot with a dog.

Sure enough, as we continued west, we came across a series of tents and tables filled with local artists. We looked through all of their work, and Peety and I wound up picking out and bartering for a gorgeous painting in colors that perfectly matched our Spanish theme. It was the first piece of original art I'd ever purchased—besides Peety's collar from Paco's, that is—and it marked the start of what would be a two-year process of putting the perfect, handmade finishing touches on our transformed home.

After loading that painting into the trunk of my car, Peety and I wandered onto a public lawn and sat there admiring the beauty of the Golden Gate Bridge.

"You know what, Peety? I've never walked that bridge. In all the years growing up here, and being back here, I've never walked the Golden Gate. I've never been to Alcatraz, either. Maybe we ought to do some of these things, you and me? What do you think? Want to walk it tomorrow?"

Peety heard the word "walk" and started spinning in circles, just raring to go.

"Not right now, boy! We've done enough. But how about tomorrow? Let's stay the night. Let's be tourists together!"

Finding a dog-friendly hotel in touristy San Francisco wasn't as easy as it was in Berkeley. Some of the big chains had a strict no-pet policy. The hotel we finally found that would let us stay the night charged an additional $100 fee. A hundred bucks! That was on top of the already overpriced room.

"Do you charge that much for people's children to join them?" I said sarcastically.

The desk clerk didn't find that amusing.

It just didn't make sense. Peety was my friend. My companion. My child in a way. I had been calling him "son" for months without even thinking about it. But he was more than that. He was my connection to the world. I needed him.

I wondered if those same hotels would have charged so much or refused service to a seeing-eye dog, or a therapy dog. And that got me thinking. I went online in the room that night and looked up the Americans with Disabilities Act (ADA). I learned that service dogs could not be excluded from hotels, restaurants, places of work, public spaces, or anywhere else. Landlords couldn't refuse to rent apartments or sell condos to people with emotional support animals or service dogs. I kept searching and found there were all sorts of different types of service dogs, from dogs that help veterans deal with the symptoms of post-traumatic stress disorder, to therapy dogs for children with autism, and dogs that help detect seizures and diabetes symptoms. It was an eye-opening moment for me to think about just how important dogs are in the lives of so many people. I had never thought about the important role they played in so many people's lives.

Peety certainly played an important role in mine. And I speculated: *I wonder if I can get approved for a service dog, so I can take Peety with me everywhere I go?*

The next morning, Peety and I set out across the Golden Gate. Step by step, we crossed one of the greatest structures ever built by man. We took our time. We stopped and gazed out over the water. We watched a giant cargo ship pass beneath us. Peety's eyes followed the path of each seagull that came swooping past us at that great height. We stopped and shared some fruit on the far side of the bridge, then made the long walk back. The entire experience was stunning.

We were tired but still raring to go. I decided we should continue our quest to be tourists for the day and take a boat out to Alcatraz. I walked Peety up to the ticket counter, and the person behind the window told me that dogs were not allowed on board.

"He's great with people. I take him everywhere," I said.

But they wouldn't budge. So we headed off to find some lunch instead. There was a Chipotle nearby, and I knew they had plant-based options that Peety and I would both enjoy, and they usually had outdoor seating where Peety could accompany me. So off we went.

"I'm sorry, son," I said. "Tell you what. I'm going to do whatever I can to make sure you can go wherever you want. We'll come back and go to Alcatraz someday soon. OK?"

I stopped and looked back at that bridge we'd crossed together. I thought about how long the walk used to be from the door of my building to the end of the block, and I simply could not believe how much our lives had changed, and how quickly.

Peety looked up at me in his brand-new collar, and in some ways, I felt like we were just getting started.

*If we could do all of that, if we could walk that giant bridge—what else can we do together?*

# chapter 13

# Get Cooking

Back home, I found a recipe on the Internet for a vegan coconut curry with sweet potatoes, turmeric, cinnamon, maple syrup, and baked tofu chunks. As the pan full of all of those wonderful fragrances heated up, Peety came running into the kitchen with his nose twitching and nostrils flaring.

"You like the smell of that?" I asked him. He started panting excitedly, wagging his tail.

"Me, too!" I said.

I took a little taste from the pan, and it was absolutely fantastic.

"Wait till you try it," I said.

I had taken to feeding him a little portion of my own plates at most meals, but on this night, Peety absolutely demanded seconds. I realized Peety might have been a little bored with the same old rice and beans and prepackaged vegan dog food he'd been eating, just as I'd become bored with the products of my limited cooking skills. I wondered what other things I might be able to make that we might really enjoy together.

"I really need to find us some cooking classes," I told him.

The very next day, Chef Philip Gelb e-mailed me back. He said the only reason he didn't use the word "vegan" on his website was because the word was a turnoff for too many people. He cooked "food," he said. Sure, it was plant-based, fresh, organic, meat- and dairy-free, but it was all "just food." He had people come to his dinners all the time who had no idea they were in for a vegan meal, he said, and he had yet to have one of those customers tell him they were unhappy or unsatisfied with the food they ate. "Good food is good food," he said.

What a great attitude.

I admired the guy already.

I went back on his website and signed up for his next class. The meal we would prepare? Paella—a Spanish rice dish that traditionally includes seafood, or a combination of chicken and various meats, including rabbit. How he'd pull that off without using any meat or animal product was beyond me, but I was excited to find out.

One task down. I had taken a step toward breaking through my food wall. Even taking that one step of signing up for the class made me feel better.

Task two? I made an appointment with a dermatologist. I needed to find a way to alleviate my plaque psoriasis. It seemed to be getting worse every day. There had to be something I could do.

Task three? I called a therapist. The difference I felt when I was with Peety as opposed to whenever I went out into the world by myself was more than troublesome. It had grown frightening. I'm not sure if it was depression, or anxiety, or a combination of both, or something else entirely, but I hated the way I felt when he wasn't with me. I realized it wasn't all that different from the way I felt on a daily basis before Peety had come into my life. I was moody. I was impatient with people at times. Mostly, I was silent. Invisible. The difference since then is I knew better. I had discovered that there was another way to live. I had experienced a taste of happiness, and joy, and connection, and bonding with another being, and I knew that I needed to be able to keep that experience going with or without Peety at my side.

I could only imagine what it would feel like to bond with a human being with anywhere near as much love and affection as I now shared with my dog. I had never done it before. Ever. And I felt it might be good to speak to a professional about whether I was doing anything to inadvertently keep myself from enjoying that possibility.

Thanks to a last-minute cancellation, I was able to get in to see the dermatologist that very same week. He took one look at the affected areas on my chest and back and said it looked like an advanced case, but he said he'd seen worse, and it was treatable with medication.

"There's one more spot," I said.

I stood up and loosened my pants. I pulled my underwear out just enough for him to take a peak down between my legs.

"You've gotta help me," I said.

"All we can do is try medication. There are a series of good medications on the market that are extremely effective for some people. It's basically just a matter of trial and error for which medication will work best for you," he said.

"So," I said, "here's the thing. I spent the last six months getting off of every medication I was on. I think you saw in my chart that I've lost more than a hundred and twenty pounds in this past year. The last thing I want to do is go on medication if I can avoid it. What I'm wondering is if it could be something in my diet that I could change, or—"

"No. There's little evidence that it's caused by diet. The good news is the medications work."

"Yeah, but what about side effects?"

"There can be side effects. No doubt. Nausea, diarrhea, and weight gain. But most patients don't experience problems, and even if they do they're fairly minor in exchange for the benefits."

"I'm not most patients. I think I've experienced every side effect of every medication I've ever been on."

"Well, let's give it a shot, and if it doesn't work, we'll try another."

The whole visit lasted less than ten minutes. He wrote me a prescription for a name-brand drug that I'd seen advertised on TV. I went so far as to go to the pharmacy to pick it up. But I couldn't take it. I just couldn't bring myself to put another drug into my system. I felt like I had finally gotten clean. The very last thing I wanted to do was swallow anything that might reverse how amazing I felt. Even a 1 percent chance of suffering those side effects seemed like too big of a chance to take.

And so the psoriasis lingered. I felt helpless.

I talked about that feeling of helplessness with the therapist I saw a week later. In fact, I talked about everything. I walked in and just let loose on her. Our first visit was supposed to be forty minutes, but I pushed it into a full hour and could have gone much longer had the next patient not been sitting in the waiting room. The therapist agreed that I was in need of help—and she agreed wholeheartedly that the biggest source of help I had in my life so far was Peety. So I asked about the concept of having Peety serve as my service dog, and much to my delight she knew what was required.

"That would require a diagnosis of a specific disability, and then the dog would have to be trained properly. It's not a minor decision, or something that's easy to do, but I would be happy to consider that option if it seems warranted," she added.

"Great!" I said. "It really would make such a difference. I know that."

She handed me a pamphlet on the process. The guidelines called for Peety to follow basic commands (which he could), and to be groomed and cared for in a way that would make him suitable to go out in public places (not a problem, thanks to my Chinese groomers), and for him to be trained to perform a specific service to help my condition. That last part seemed like a potential snag. What specific service did Peety provide? I didn't have a diagnosed condition, except for obesity, and I already knew that wasn't considered a disability under ADA guidelines. The thought that I could maybe someday have the ability to take Peety with me everywhere I went was comforting. But I walked out of her office that day thinking it was probably nothing more than a pipe dream.

I was surprised to find Chef Philip's studio in a gritty part of town. He was set up in a brick, former factory-type building where a variety of artists and musicians apparently found affordable studio space. At first I was a little nervous leaving my car on the street and wondered if maybe I'd made a bad decision.

Once I stepped inside, though, all of my concerns disappeared.

There were three other people there for the class already, and I was the last to arrive. Every one of those people greeted me with a great big smile, a glass of wine in their hand, and a warm, welcoming "hello." Chef Philip had light-brown hair pulled back into a ponytail, and there was nothing about his kitchen that was fancy or exclusive or pretentious. He had a basic electric coil-top stove and a couple of stainless-steel worktables. His pots and pans didn't shine like new. They carried the patina of well-worn tools. The space was clean but not well organized. It seemed like I was stepping into the office of a genius professor, or maybe a mad scientist. The fridge was basic and covered with magnets and stickers. A rice cooker and a Crock-Pot were plugged in around a corner on a makeshift table, next to a music stand and some sheet music. The dining table was plain dark wood.

He did have a fantastic looking ice cream–making machine off to one side—a stainless-steel Italian gelato maker that he said could freeze a raw cashew-based "ice cream" dessert in half the time of most ice cream makers, and perhaps we'd have time to try it out at the end of the night. And he had an industrial blender unlike anything I'd ever seen. It looked like the type of blender you'd see in a high-priced smoothie shop, with a black, rubbery looking base and a tall, squared off plastic chamber, but it was twice as wide, in addition to being well worn and heavily used.

As someone put a glass of wine in my hand (noting that it was vegan), I could smell the fresh herbs spread out on the center worktable.

Chef Philip handed around a photocopy of a hand-written recipe with the ingredients and measurements of his signature paella all listed out. He told us all to grab a knife and get chopping. He came around and helped us with our knife techniques, telling the one young woman in the class to curl her fingers under her knuckles so she wouldn't chop them off as she pushed an onion toward the blade. I thought it looked a lot like the fist-like gesture I'd been told to make when I first met Peety. Meanwhile, I got busy chopping some cilantro, and some "culantro," which was a tropical variant he said that had a slightly different flavor. He ripped off a piece and sniffed it and chewed it, and I did the same. I was still surprised by how one tiny leaf of one herb could fill up my senses so completely.

We were off and running, and it soon became clear that everyone in that room was there for the very same reason: to expand their knowledge and skills in plant-based cuisine.

My classmates had all become vegans for different reasons. One man suffered from bad food allergies all his life and saw them disappear once he removed all animal products from his diet. The woman, who was in her twenties, said she could just no longer stomach the idea of eating animals. She looked at them and knew they had feelings. All of them, she said. She just couldn't stand to eat them anymore, or to see them "abused" by being penned up in factory farms.

"Have you ever driven that stretch of I-Five—"

"With the stench," Chef Philip said.

We all moaned in agreement. We had all driven that stretch. Anyone who's ever traveled up or down I-5 between San Francisco and LA has encountered that stench. Locally it was known as "the big stink."

"Yeah. Those giant herds of cows lining up for the slaughter. It's just the most foul smell of death and—"

"Manure," one of the men said.

"Yeah," I agreed. "It's awful."

"Honestly, I can't drive that way anymore," she said. "I'll go hours out of my way just to avoid it. Seeing those herds, knowing all of those thousands of animals are just waiting in the hot sun to be taken to slaughter. It's like driving through the Auschwitz of cows."

That phrase stuck in my mind like fried chicken used to stick in my gut. I hadn't done a whole lot of thinking about the ethical or animal-rights side of a plant-based diet, and that discussion hit me like a slap in the face.

"They're creatures just as we are," Chef Philip chimed in. "My turning point was when I was off visiting a farm property with some friends after college, and there was this one cow that came ambling over to my friend as we were sitting by the pond. The cow came all the way out there to find her, and then laid down next to her and put her head on my friend's lap. She sat there petting it, and that cow had this unbelievable look of contentment on her face. It was exactly what a dog might do, and I just thought, 'How can we kill these things for *food* when we're surrounded by acres and acres of foods we can eat without having to kill anything at all?'"

The third guy agreed with the woman and Chef Philip, but he argued that the environmental reason for choosing a plant-based diet was the most important reason of all. I sort of tuned out as he was talking because I was stuck on the image of that cow with its head on a girl's lap in a beautiful sunny field by a pond. I pictured Peety with his head on my lap as he looked up at me with that familiar look of adoration in his eyes, and I shivered.

I didn't expect to ever go back to eating meat again, just because of how much better I felt after giving it up. But somehow, I thought, *The imagery of that happy cow—along with my personal memories of the stench on I-5—may very well keep me from eating meat ever again, no matter what temptation I face in the future.*

As we dug into the finer preparations of the meal, we shared our mutual stories of early failures in the kitchen. Each of us, Chef Philip included, had overcooked broccoli the first time they steamed it. Every one of us had burned rice on the stove. Every one of us had gone a little overboard after we found the joy of using exotic spices and then combined way too many spices in a single dish.

"Sometimes a little salt and pepper on a perfectly cooked vegetable is all you need. It's perfection," Chef Philip said.

That's when I brought up a method of cooking called

steam frying—a technique that puts an end to the need for cooking with oil. I'd found it online and taught myself by watching YouTube videos. "The primary reason people cook with oil is because it doesn't evaporate as you're cooking," I said. "But you can accomplish the same thing with water. You just add a little water to your frying pan or wok, and just keep adding water back as it evaporates. So as it boils out, you add more, and that boiling action keeps the food from sticking to the pan the same as oil does, with a fraction of the calories."

"I've tried it," Chef Gelb said. "It's not for me, in most cases, because I'm not looking to cut calories. I'm cooking for flavor and texture and enjoyment. But I agree that it works great, and if you need to cut calories, it's a great method."

"It's especially useful when you're cooking something like potatoes," I said. "I love breakfast potatoes, right? But if you cook them with oil, you start out with some oil, and that oil gets absorbed, and so you wind up adding a little more oil to the pan, and before you know it you've tripled the calories. If you just eat the potatoes without that oil, they are just as filling and satisfying but with a fraction of the calories."

"Yeah, but I like potatoes crispy. You can't do that without oil," the woman said.

"Actually, just last week I tried steaming them first and really making them soft, then baking, and I swear to you they were brown and crispy on the outside and soft on the inside, even though they were healthier they tasted even better without all of that grease and oil."

"That's cool," Chef Philip said. "Finding what you love

and what works for you is the key to cooking. Don't be afraid to keep trying new things until you get it right."

As a group, we lamented the lack of good vegan cheese in the world. That was something we all missed. There were good vegan spreading cheeses starting to come on the market, and most were made from cultured cashews and other nuts. But melting a slice of cheese for a grilled-cheese sandwich still seemed like an unattainable vegan dream. "But eventually somebody will figure it out. We're making all kinds of things now, with all sorts of textures and flavors that people thought were impossible to achieve without dairy," Chef Philip said.

That thought got him started on a new recipe for cashew-based "ice cream" again, and he insisted we all had to try it. So he pulled out a plastic bin full of raw cashews and tossed them into his industrial-looking blender with some water, whipping them into a frothy smooth liquid that looked like heavy cream. He threw in some agave syrup for sweetness, added some blueberries, and tossed the mixture into the Italian contraption.

"Wait till you try this," he said.

The fact that nuts and soybeans and coconut and so many things could be turned into "milk" was still amazing to me. And seeing how he turned nuts into liquid in his own kitchen so quickly made me think, *I need to buy one of those blenders!*

"Maybe one of *you* will come up with the solution for a melting vegan cheese one day," he said. "The coolest innovations are often invented by accident or through trial and error in home kitchens like this one."

One of the things that I found most impressive in Chef Philip's kitchen was that nothing came prepackaged. Not one thing. The man made his own tofu. He ground his own spices and curries from whole plants using a mortar and pestle.

I never realized just how much that attention to detail could matter.

The paella we ate that night was better than anything I'd ever tasted, including any non-vegan meal I'd consumed at the finest restaurants in any city I'd ever traveled to on an expense account for work. The flavors and textures and richness of pure food, from the earth, made from scratch, entirely from fresh ingredients, was the difference between the sound of a Stradivarius violin and the "violin" sound on a twenty-dollar Casio keyboard. It was the difference between listening to the Beatles on an old AM radio and experiencing an analog playback of the original *Sgt. Pepper's* reel-to-reel tapes through the finest stereo system on the planet. I'm making these music analogies because Chef Philip is also a musician, and just from the way he spoke I could tell he cared about music and the quality of sound and craftsmanship in the concert hall as much as he cared about his food. Listening to him speak, watching him move about the room, throw spices into that industrial-strength blender, cook the rice to chewy-crispy perfection in a giant paella pan, and then sit down and close his eyes as he marveled at the flavors of it all right alongside us was an absolute lesson in passion and inspiration. I wanted to bring that level of passion to every meal I made. More than that, I wanted to share this food with everyone I knew. I wanted to become truly great at this so I could share this experience with others, and maybe have a shot at inspiring other people in the world to try this life-style I'd now embraced so fully, and so easily.

I would make plans to attend every Chef Philip course I could in the coming months. He and I would become friends. He invited me to call or e-mail with questions any-time I wanted, and he was always happy to engage in a dis-cussion about food. He turned me onto bigger, better, more interesting markets in the region that carried more vegeta-bles in one room than I'd ever seen in my life. He shared stories about the death of old farms that had been taken over by modern-day industrial food-growth methods, which were later reclaimed by new food pioneers who returned the soil and the trees to their former glory—unlocking fruits and vegetables that were so filled once again with their natural, bountiful flavors that customers came flocking, in droves.

Talking to a man like Philip Gelb, it's hard not to walk away and want to do everything you can to change the world. And taking that first cooking class with him unlocked a pas-sion for cooking in me that I hoped would never, ever go away.

# chapter 14

# Milestones

I want it to go away," I said. "I can't stand it. I don't know what to do."

My first monthly visit back to Dr. Preeti immediately took a turn away from anything to do with my weight loss. That part of my life was fine. Peety was doing great. I told her all about our walk over the Golden Gate and how much Peety was enjoying his newly expanded variety of vegan dishes, thanks to my new skills in the kitchen. Plus, I had continued to drop up to five pounds per week without putting any additional effort in at all.

But the plaque psoriasis, including the patch on my privates, had grown unbearable.

"I don't know what it is. Everything about me feels better. I'm eating healthy. I've cut most sugars now. I've cut out all of the oil in my cooking. I just feel like this rash is being caused by something I'm eating, Dr. Preeti. It's grown worse, much worse since I've started eating this way. I don't understand it. All of Peety's skin problems, his itching, flaking, all of it, went away when I switched him to vegan dog food."

"OK," she said. "So. You think it's linked to food. That's your instinct. Have you thought about environmental factors, including any chemicals in laundry detergents?" she asked.

"I read that somewhere, yes. I switched to a hypoallergenic laundry detergent a while ago. It made no difference. I suppose my dry cleaning could be a problem. I could try to find an all-natural dry cleaner, but I hate to take business away from the guy I go to. He's a buddy now. Plus, my underwear doesn't get dry-cleaned. Why would I have it *there*?"

"I think the best thing you can do is try an elimination diet. Cut your diet down to just a few foods—plain rice, some fruit—for a few days and see if any of the symptoms subside. Assuming they do, then try adding foods back one at a time, very slowly, and keeping track of what you eat. It will be tedious, but that's the only way you're going to know if this is being caused by a reaction to something in your diet."

"I'll do it. I'll do anything. I can't take it anymore," I said.

I cut my diet back to nothing but plain rice and green peas for the next two days. I added in some peaches and bananas for vitamins, and I stuck to that for a few days. It was tough. I was coming off of the biggest cooking renaissance I'd ever experienced. I replicated Chef Philip's paella in my own kitchen and even modified it a bit to make it my own. I figured out how to make scrambled tofu "eggs" that tasted even better than the ones I enjoyed at the Berkeley café. I made breakfast potatoes that were out of this world!

To suddenly put all of that on hold felt like a punishment. But I needed to do this. I was so close to feeling like a normal human being. So close!

Over the course of the next four weeks, I added foods slowly. One at a time. Potatoes. Tofu. Broccoli, carrots, and various fruits. My psoriasis was nearly gone by the third week. It was astounding. I had absolutely no doubt that it was a reaction to food at that point, and I was determined to figure out which food was the culprit. One night, just for a change of scenery, I went out to one of the little Mexican joints that Mario had recommended to me. I ordered up some veggie tacos on corn tortillas. They knew how I liked it. They prepared it without any unknown ingredients. I was certain of that. And in the morning, I woke up with a newly inflamed patch of plaque psoriasis on my elbow.

I went back through the ingredients of the tacos in my mind. Every vegetable in it was something I had already eaten in the past three weeks. I was sure of that. The only thing I hadn't touched in all of that time was corn. *Corn!*

I had a package of flash-frozen corn in the freezer. I pulled it out, boiled it up, and ate a bowl of it for breakfast. Then I air-popped some popcorn in my microwave and ate the entire bowl. By the end of that day, the psoriasis on my elbow was worse, and another patch of it showed up on my chest. I was itching horribly.

Ever since I had switched to a plant-based diet, corn had become one of my go-to foods. It was a sweet and colorful addition to a stir-fry. It was a perfect, easy-to-make side dish. It tasted great on the cob with just a little salt, cooked al dente, or grilled and bursting with flavor. At all of those restaurants, it was the perfect wheat-free wrap for my tacos and burritos and all of the other Mexican delights I'd come to cherish.

Corn.

I cut it out completely and resumed the rest of my now-regular diet, and a week later, when I went to see Dr. Preeti for my monthly follow-up, I walked in with a big smile on my face.

"I got it," I said. "I found the culprit."

Dr. Preeti wasn't one to show much emotion, but when I told her the psoriasis was gone, she clapped her hands together and let out a little "Whoop!" of a cheer. "I'm so happy to hear that!"

I hopped on the scale and found myself faced with even more good news. I had broken two hundred pounds. I checked in at 198. I hadn't weighed less than two hundred pounds since shortly after I got out of the army.

I was now less than twenty pounds from my goal weight.

"I'm actually going to make it," I said.

"I think you are, yes."

"I mean...it's not even a question. There's no reason not to. My body has been taking care of itself on its own, doing this on its own. I'm just feeding it what it wants to be fed, and that's it."

"That's certainly been the case so far. And it can continue to be the case. But it can also get tricky from here. Once you hit your goal weight, you may find it harder to keep the weight off. Many people have a tendency to become complacent and backslide once they achieve a weight loss goal, such as stopping workouts and eating foods that caused their obesity and health problems in the first place," Dr. Preeti said.

"What can I do? I don't want that to happen," I said.

"I think it's still important that you find some more social activity. I'm so happy to hear about the cooking classes, but I mean something more like a runner's group, or a biking group, or something outdoors and athletic. You don't like the gym, if I recall, but a swim club, or something. Your body will crave some sort of activity that's a little more rigorous, and it's important that you find some sort of exercise that you don't hate. If you can find an activity you actually like, one that you do with other people, you'll find maintaining your results to be much easier."

"Ah," I said. "Yeah. OK. Well, so far I've done my best to do everything you suggest, so I'll try to do this, too. It won't be easy. But I'll try."

Just over one month later, I hopped on my digital bathroom scale and found I was down to 180 pounds. Ever since I'd broken down and bought that scale, I'd marveled at how often the weight on that scale had been consistent with what I weighed on Dr. Preeti's scale. The laws of physics weren't different in the doctor's office after all. Somehow, in the past, I had just been fooling myself into thinking I weighed five or ten pounds less than I actually did. I didn't own a digital scale before. Maybe the old scale was off. Or maybe, just maybe, I tilted my head in a way that made the needle look like it was landing on a different line.

So much of how we see the world is what we make of it in our minds.

"Well, Peety, what do you think of that?" I said.

He looked up at me from the bathroom floor like, *"Yeah. So what? When are we going to get out of here and go outside?!"*

Whenever I'd hit a weight-loss goal in the past, at Weight Watchers meetings or anywhere else, there was a celebration. "Hooray! Woo-hoo!" Even if I was by myself, I'd feel like partying. I'd treat myself to a prize of some sort, a purchase maybe, or a dinner at a really nice restaurant. But life isn't like an episode of *The Biggest Loser*. Weight loss isn't a competition. It's not a one-time accomplishment. Hitting 180 wasn't the goal. Feeling healthy, being healthy, feeling "normal," being able to walk without pain, being able to live without pain and feel good—those were the goals. And those were ongoing goals. It didn't feel like winning. It felt like I could breathe a sigh of relief. As if now—finally—I could get started on the rest of my life.

I knew with everything in my heart that I was never going to regain that weight again. So I went out wardrobe shopping—this time with the intention to keep everything I bought for a long time. I'd purchased new clothes about every six weeks over the course of the past ten months. I tossed all of those transitional garments into black plastic trash bags and hauled them off to Goodwill. I walked into Macy's and bought some pants and shirts I knew I would be able to keep. I also went to the mall and stepped foot into an athletic store. I purchased new workout clothes. I bought some new sneakers—in addition to losing the girth around my midsection, I had dropped a shoe size and a half, plus two full widths.

The only "sport" I had ever really participated in since

kickball in grade school was running, and that was only because I was forced to do it in the army. I had no interest in running, and I hadn't so much as jogged more than a few feet with Peety during all of our many walks together—and only then when we had to cross a street quickly or needed to move away from the path of another dog he kept barking at.

As I thought about Dr. Preeti's advice, though, and my desire to follow it, I couldn't think of anything else I even remotely wanted to do. I didn't own a bike, and I didn't feel like shopping for one. I had little interest in swimming. I still hated the gym. What else was there to do?

"Some of my patients have tried Zumba," Dr. Preeti told me, "including some who hated the gym, and once they were in a class with all of those other people, dancing, having a good time, they realized they wanted to come back. They didn't want to quit."

I was pretty sure *Zumba* wasn't going to be my thing. I knew I had no natural rhythm. My style of dancing involved repeatedly bending my knees, and when I did that in front of Peety once, he barked at me.

So early one evening, just after the hot sun went down but while there was still some light in the sky, I popped Peety into the backseat and we drove down to the old San Jose State University running track. That track had been quite a place in its day. Some legendary runners had trained there. Runners who won gold medals at the Olympics in the 1960s. The track was all neglected and pitted now. In more recent decades, the university had sunk its resources into building a football team and a stadium to go with it. They used that legendary old track mostly as a parking lot now for the minor league ballpark across the street. But it was still there.

I parked my car in the middle and rolled the windows down so Peety would be comfortable. I got out, stretched a little bit, and stood on that track in my new running shoes, shorts, and a shirt that was supposed to be made of a new-fangled breathable material to whisk away sweat. I thought, *This is crazy.*

But then I took a deep breath and got to it. I started at a slow pace, just to see how it felt. I saw Peety watching me, switching from one side of the car to the other as I rounded the track, just so he could keep an eye on me. I could tell he thought I was crazy, too. *What the heck is my dad doing?!*

The track was a quarter mile around, and I found that I made it around the whole thing pretty easily that first time. My legs carried me fine. My knees felt good. The new shoes were awesome. I wasn't breathing too hard. I decided to pick up the pace a little bit, and once I found a stride, it felt like my body was almost carrying itself along. My legs moved in straight lines. No more swinging. No more "thump, thump, thump." I seemed to almost bounce back up into the air every time a foot hit the ground, as if my legs were expecting me to weigh more than I did and were automatically over-compensating.

My breathing got heavier, and I could feel my heart pumping, but I came around for a second full lap, and I felt like I could keep going.

It was kind of astounding to think about the fact that I'd carried almost double my weight for so many years. My legs had been carrying an extra hundred and fifty pounds, day in and day out. I suppose that must have built up some muscles over the years. I supposed all the walking I'd done with Peety had helped get my legs in shape, too, because this actually felt kind of good. I was huffing and puffing pretty hard as I looped around for a third time. A streetlight flickered on as I heard the night sounds of crickets, and a warm California breeze blew in from the west. Something in me told me to keep going.

"Woof!" Peety barked, watching intently as I ran by, with his head extending outside the car window. "Woof, woof!"

I ran harder, just to see if I could. And I *could*. I pushed and pushed and came around the final bend feeling nearly out of breath. But I did it. I completed an entire mile on that track, running as fast as I could for the entire last lap.

I slowed my body down and put my hands on my hips, bending over to catch my breath. I was drenched with sweat.

"Woof-woof-woof-woof," Peety barked.

"I'm OK, boy!" I shouted. "I'm good, I'm good." I waved at him as I felt my elevated heart rate slow down to something approaching normal in less than a minute.

I walked back to the car and grabbed a towel off the passenger seat as Peety licked my face. He liked the taste of all that extra salt on my cheeks. I wiped the sweat and Peety slobber from my forehead and took Peety out and walked him around slowly as my body cooled down. He seemed to feed off of my energy. He tugged at the leash, pulling me forward.

"You want to try running with me next time?" I asked him.

I could hardly believe those words when I said them:

"Next time." I actually thought, *Yeah, I should try this again. I bet I could go two miles if I didn't push so hard.*

I came back to the track the next night and tried to run with Peety, but he wasn't interested. He kept trying to bite the leash or pull us off the track to go sniff something.

I put him in the backseat to watch me again and promised we'd take a walk afterward. Then I went back to the starting line and began. I ran a total of eight laps, which was two full miles, and neither my knees nor my feet hurt. So I vowed to come back.

I returned again the next night. This time I ran three miles. It astounded me that I could do that without doing anything special to prepare for it. Had I inadvertently been training myself for the entire time I'd been slimming down?

I took Peety on a victory lap around the track, walking that quarter mile instead of running. He sniffed at every pot-hole and crack, and seemed to approve. He seemed to walk with pride on that new surface, mirroring the pride that I felt in what I had accomplished.

It was as if my body had warmed up with every mile I ran and prepared itself to run a little farther the next time, just in case. It felt as if my body could do almost anything I wanted it to do.

That's all it took. Three runs. I decided that running might be my thing. I went out the next day and invested in a pair of New Balance running shoes.

Now, I just needed to add the social component.

So I went online and found a number of South Bay Area meet-up groups dedicated to running. Some were for serious hard-core marathon and triathlon types. Those weren't for me. But there were others dedicated to recreational runners, beginners, people who wanted to try to get into shape. So I focused on those.

One of those groups happened to be headed up by a very attractive brunette named Sarah. She seemed like a really active leader. She kept a blog about the group, and it all seemed very relaxed and open. As I read about their upcoming activities, I kept looking back at her profile picture and thinking, *Wow. That woman is stunning!*

Of all the groups I could have decided to join, I thought, *Why not pick that one?*

I sent Sarah a note, and she wrote back the same night.

"Sure! Come join us this Sunday," she wrote. "Would love to have you. Oh, and spread the word. We're always looking for new members. Bring friends!"

It's a pretty cold feeling to see the word "friends" and realize you don't really have any to speak of. I had clients and business friends from the appliance stores I called on, but I didn't hang out with any of them outside of work. I knew Mario the barber, the dog groomers, and my dry cleaner. And Sally my housekeeper who did excellent work. I got along great with Dr. Preeti. I had the old lady on the stoop down around the block I said hello to sometimes. And I had Peety. That was it.

I really hoped that was about to change.

# chapter 15

# Sarah Smile

One month later, I did the math in my head as I looked in the mirror trying to figure out what new shirt to wear with my brand-new jeans. *How can it be fifteen years since I've done this?*

I wasn't even really sure if I could call it a date. It was a play date—for our dogs. It was a chance to talk about the plans we'd devised to throw a vegan dinner party for some members of our running group who seemed genuinely interested in changing their diets, and changing their lives. Yet we planned to meet at Sarah's house, just the two of us. I'd promised to cook a fabulous vegan dinner for her, and I couldn't help but think that all of our post-run talks over coffee were kind of flirtatious. *Weren't they?*

I didn't want to try too hard. I didn't want to dress up too much and make her think I was presuming this was anything more than friendship mixed with business mixed with our mutual love of dogs, but I really, really wanted to impress her. The only times she'd seen me, ever since our very first encounter at the head of the Los Gatos Creek Trail, I'd been dressed in workout clothes, all sweaty and salt encrusted. That was the only way I'd seen her, too. Still, I couldn't help but fantasize about what she might look like with her hair let down from her ponytail.

It was still hard for me to fathom how my life could have changed so quickly. In the course of a single month since hitting my goal weight, I had transformed into a social person. Peety had transformed, too. We had play dates with other people's dogs. And for some reason, he seemed to understand implicitly that my friend's dogs weren't the enemy. He never barked at them when they first met. He still barked at strangers' dogs on our walks. But never my friends' dogs, as long as we first met them outside rather than at the door of Peety's castle. It was wild.

The idea of having a beer or a glass of wine while our dogs ran around in the backyard was something entirely new to me. It was an excuse to socialize, and Peety approached every one of those moments with a look of adventure and kindness in his eyes.

It's as if the two of us were ugly trolls who'd finally emerged from under a bridge.

Only four people showed up to my first meet-up group run. Me and three others: Vicki, Chris, and group-leader Sarah. Sarah was even more attractive in person than she was in her profile pic, and it was all I could do not to stare at the ground in her presence. She seemed way out of my league. I didn't even know if she was single. I felt foolish for showing up and thinking that this woman might show some interest in me.

I'd never done a trail run before, and I told them I was nervous right at the start. They were all friendly, and sympathetic, and said they'd take it easy on me. I told them I'd only started running that week, and they were all so encouraging. I fell behind after the first couple of miles, but Vicki was kind enough to hold back and chat with me while I struggled, and that really kept me going. I told her a little bit about the journey I'd been on over the course of the last year, and when we met the others at the end of the trail, she insisted we all go to breakfast so I could tell them my full story.

I was astounded at how interested these three fit, professional people were in hearing my tale of woe and the long, winding road to recovery. They seemed to hang on every word, as if it was the most interesting story they'd ever heard. They laughed at my memories of Peety jumping into the pond, and my first encounters with Mario the barber, and my stories about shopping and feeling miserable every time I saw myself in the dressing-room mirrors. They kept saying things like, "I cannot believe you weighed over three hundred pounds," and "You'd never know it to look at you now," and "There's no way you're fifty-two! Stop it. You're lying!"

Over the course of that first conversation, I found out that Sarah was divorced and unattached. But the thought of even the possibility of asking her out completely terrified me. So I didn't do it. Instead, I engaged her in discussions about my new industrial-strength blender and the incredible smoothies I made at breakfast now that gave me all the nutrition I needed to feel like Superman.

That first run turned into a weekly event at a different location each week. More runners joined in. Some others set up weekday early-morning runs, and I joined in some of those, too, after getting Peety up and out extra early for our regular thirty-minute walks every morning on top of it all. Peety really loved his walks, and I could not deprive him of them—our outside time together kept us both close no matter how much busier my life became.

Our group often went for coffee or breakfast afterward, and each time we did, I wound up sitting right next to Sarah. After the third time we wound up next to each other, it no longer seemed like a coincidence. I loved her confidence and her enthusiasm for running. Everyone who joined that group just seemed filled with passion and joy. These were exactly the type of people I wanted to be around, and they seemed to think I fit right in.

They all loved hearing about the adventurous side of my diet, and how I'd learned all sorts of new recipes from Chef Philip, and pretty soon they started asking if I could share recipes or show them how to cook some of this fabulous new food themselves. They were just so blown away by the results of my transformation that nearly everyone in the group wondered what going vegan—even for a few meals a week— might do for their own health and fitness.

"I'm positive it will help you feel younger and stronger than you've ever felt before," I said. "But if you want the full-blown effects, you've got to go all the way. This isn't something that works by going partway. Cut out the animal foods, and watch what happens. Within a week, I bet you'll feel like a new person."

I realized I was becoming an advocate, a vocal proponent for what Dr. Preeti had taught me.

One day, as I described my modified Chef Philip recipe for vegan paella in mouthwatering detail, Sarah said, "That's it. You need to have us all over for dinner," and everyone at the table said, "Yes! Please! Let's do that!"

I looked at her adorable smile and without even thinking about it I replied, "That would be great!"

Sarah, being the go-getter she was, decided to kick it up a notch. She started brainstorming all sorts of ideas for this party and how we could make it something more. She wondered if maybe everyone could chip in a little something, and we could use the dinner party as a fund-raiser for an animal shelter or welfare organization. It turned out she had a dog that she loved, too, a big golden-doodle named Daisy. We decided we needed much more time to plan it all and talk about it, and that morphed into the plans that had me running to the nearest Macy's for some date-night clothes and hurrying to get dressed so I could swing by the farmer's market on the way to her house.

Peety lay on the bed behind me, watching with keen interest as I tore off the blue shirt and tried on a black V-neck tee that I wasn't sure would fit. It was a *medium*. I hadn't worn a size medium anything in as long as I could remember. It was a little tight through the chest as I pulled it on. The sleeves were a little tight, too, and the feeling of that stretchy fabric on my skin felt strange—but compared to the large shirts I'd been trying, the tightness of it actually looked good. It surprised me to look in the mirror. That shirt, which felt far too small to me, didn't look too small at all. In fact, it accentuated my muscles.

It turned out I had developed a surprisingly good physique under all of that fat, perhaps just from the workout of carrying all of that fat around every day. Now that I was running and had burned off a little extra layer of body fat, those muscles were *visible*. And *defined*.

"Look at that, Peety," I said. "What do you think?"

Peety's ears perked up. He cocked his head to the side.

"Can I really pull this off?" I asked him.

He started panting with excitement and flashed me a big doggie smile. I took that as a thumbs-up.

"All right, boy. Let's go!" I said, and down he jumped, circling my legs like a puppy. He clearly knew this night was something special, too.

With my arms full of grocery bags, I rang Sarah's doorbell with my elbow, and my heart started pounding like a teenager's. Peety heard the barking inside and kept looking at me, wondering what he was about to find on the other side of that door. Finally, it opened, and there Sarah stood: her dark hair brushing her shoulders, framing her gorgeous face, all fresh and beautiful with just a touch of makeup. She looked incredible. She was dressed in a nice shirt and jeans, just like me, and it was clear that she'd put some thought into getting ready, too. I could tell right away that my instincts had been right: this get-together was more than just professional and potentially more than "just friends."

"Hi!" she said, first to Peety, squatting down to scratch behind his ears. "And hi to you, too," she said, standing up and taking one of the grocery bags from me. Her golden-doodle Daisy was bouncing all over the place behind her, and Peety was practically dancing, just itching to go inside. "Go ahead, boy," I said, letting go of his leash.

"Hi," I said to Sarah.

"Come on in," she said, leading us into the kitchen. Peety and Daisy were jumping around so much they kept bumping into the furniture, and us.

"Hi, Daisy," I said as I set the groceries down. I tried to pet her but she was way too excited by Peety's presence to pay any attention to me.

"Maybe we should let them into the backyard to burn off some energy," Sarah said with a laugh.

"That's probably a good idea."

I loved how relaxed she was about the dogs' hyperactivity.

"Does anything need to go in the fridge?" she asked me.

"No, no, it's all from the farmer's market. It's fine on the counter," I said.

"Can I get you something to drink?" she asked as she opened the back door.

"Yeah, sure," I said. "I could go for some chardonnay if you have it."

"Chardonnay's my favorite!" she said as I scooted by her to follow the dogs at the same time she stepped inside toward the kitchen.

Peety and Daisy started chasing each other around. It was a sizable fenced-in yard for San Jose, with an impressive twisting garden of watermelon vines growing along one fence.

"I take it you like watermelons," I called toward the door.

"My daughter and her friends threw a bunch of seeds

there, and they grew into this. Isn't it wild?" she called back.

"It's awesome!" I answered.

Peety's inner border collie came out as he kept trying to pin Daisy down, but she kept breaking away from him, teasing him, almost laughing at him, looking back over her shoulder as she ran away over and over again. It was hilarious to watch.

"Wow. I guess they're getting along just fine," Sarah said, handing me a glass.

"Yeah, I should say so," I responded.

"Cheers," she said, smiling and tipping her glass toward mine. I looked her in the eyes and smiled back as I clinked her glass. The night was off to a better start than I could have imagined.

It felt strange to have any sort of confidence. It felt strange to walk into that house with some swagger. Those feelings still fit loosely, like an oversized shirt. But I wanted to tailor them and wear them well, and Sarah seemed to make that easy.

"You know," I said as we walked back in to make dinner, "I was doing the math before I came over, and I realized I haven't been on a date in, like, fifteen years."

"Oh, man," Sarah said. "I know *that* feeling."

In Sarah's case, she knew what it felt like to be single again after a long relationship, but I also knew she was very aware of what had kept me off the market for so long. I felt like a fool. I suddenly felt fat again. My stomach twisted up in a knot. I started unpacking the veggies and hoped she might change the subject.

"So," she said, reaching into one of the bags and pulling out a big, fresh, deep-red heirloom tomato. "Is this a date?"

My face must've turned that same shade, because she seemed very amused.

"Ummm…" I said. My mouth seemed unable to form words.

"Because I was kinda hoping this was a date, too," she said.

I let out a big sigh. "Oh, thank God!" I said, and we both laughed.

Sarah tipped the bag over, ever so gently, and spread all of those beautiful, colorful tomatoes on her counter. We looked at each other in silence for a moment, and I felt my nerves melt into something entirely different. I wasn't exactly sure what that feeling was at first. I didn't recognize it. But slowly, as she washed the tomatoes and handed them to me, one by one, the realization began to set in.

We were connecting.

And it felt *good*.

Every time she looked at me and smiled it felt like I was dreaming. I kept asking myself, *Is this really happening?*

Within a couple of hours we were snuggled up on her couch to watch a movie together. A few minutes into it, she turned and draped her legs over mine. I ran my fingers gently, timidly, up and down the length of her jeans, and she responded, "Mmmmm."

She touched my forearm and pulled my hand up to her waist.

Neither one of us was looking at the screen anymore.

I was still shy. Still looking down. She put her hand gently under my chin and lifted my face to look me in the eye. I smiled and let out a little nervous laugh. She was just so beautiful. She bit her lip as she smiled at me, and she looked down at my mouth, and I just couldn't help myself. I leaned in, gently squeezing her waist, and kissed her. Her lips were so warm, and soft, and she wrapped her arm around the back of my neck and pulled me closer. My whole body tingled with sensations I hadn't felt in as long as I could remember. She kissed me harder, and my whole body came alive. I slid my hand down onto her thigh and pulled my legs up onto the couch. She rolled over with ease to make room for me right next to her on those narrow cushions, wrapping her legs in mine as I kissed her neck.

"Oh, God," she whispered. I could feel her hips pull in to mine, and I kissed her neck with abandon, wrapping my arms around her tiny frame and squeezing her to me.

"You are so beautiful," I whispered between kisses. "I can't believe this. I just can't—"

"Shhhh," she said. "I want you. I want you so much."

"I want you, too."

She kissed me passionately and pressed every inch of her body into mine as her hand slid down my back and over my hips and grasped my thigh.

"Maybe we should move this into the bedroom," she whispered.

I pulled my face back just enough to see her expression. Her hair fell across her face as her fingers intertwined with mine, and in that moment, I was sure she was the sexiest woman I had ever seen. I looked into her eyes and every ounce of doubt and insecurity I still carried melted away.

I pulled my legs out from under her, sitting myself up as I kissed her, and I held her hand. I stood up as she lay there with her hand still in mine, still looking at me with that incredible look of desire and passion. I felt every inch of my body, alive and filled with intensity all the way out to my fingertips and the tips of my toes, and I knew: I was ready. I was fifteen years' worth of pent-up, tamped-down, held-back ready!

I reached my left arm under her shoulders and my right arm under her knees, and I swept her up into my arms. She wrapped her arms around my neck and kissed me again as I held her in the air, and I carried her off into the dimly lit, candle-scented confines of her room.

I don't think there's a tape measure long enough to measure the smile on my face when I woke the next morning all tangled up under the covers with that woman. Sarah gave me what was easily one of the greatest nights in my entire life. A drenching rainstorm after fifteen years of drought. She was gentle and kind, and passionate and fiery at the same. It was like my first time all over again, only now with the experience and knowledge of everything we wish we knew when we were young, combined with the energy and passion of feeling better in my own body than I'd ever felt in my life.

The moment Sarah got out of bed, Peety jumped right up into her spot and put his head on her pillow.

"Ha! I think he's jealous!" Sarah laughed.

"It's OK, boy," I said, scratching Peety behind the ears. "Your dad's a happy guy!"

Sarah and I let our dogs out together and watched them run around in the yard again over coffee. I was thrilled to find some tofu in her fridge, and I wowed her with my breakfast scramble and what she called the most "amazing" breakfast potatoes she'd ever tasted.

My body tingled all over as we kept touching each other all through breakfast, and as Peety snuggled his warm coat up to my feet under the table, I remember thinking I could not have wished for anything more in the world.

It seemed impossible that just one year earlier—one year, almost to the day—I had wished and prayed for my life to come to an end.

With my body and mind experiencing a high unlike anything I had ever known, light-years beyond the high of any drug or anything else I had ever consumed, I thanked God the whole way home. I thanked God for answering my prayer.

He *had* taken my life. He saw to it that I put that miserable old me in the grave. He made me reborn. He gave me a new life in place of my old life. He sent me the signs and the angels I needed to find my way to a life of happiness that I now firmly believed was not only possible, but achievable for any person on this planet. At fifty-two years old, I was finally *living*, fully, as a loving, passionate, connected human being. If I, of all people, could get there in a year, I could only begin to imagine how many others could get there if they asked for the help and followed the signs and guidance of the earthly angels around them.

Of course, in my case, the greatest angel of all was the one who kept panting in my ear as I drove home; the one who was right there with me, encouraging me, getting me outside, taking me out of my pent-up head and gently forcing me to think of something besides my own misery, while loving me unconditionally every step of the way—even when I felt unlovable.

As I lay in my own bed that night with no one but Peety snuggled up next to me, I said right out loud, hoping God would hear me: "Thank you for giving me this amazing dog."

# chapter 16

# The Social Network

Sarah and I were interlocked in a relationship for the next six months. A perfectly normal, mostly healthy, adult relationship. I fell head-over-heels for her. In fact, I may have gone a bit overboard. That's understandable, right? After so many years of going without, it's only natural that we might have a tendency to over-indulge the first person who shows us any affection. And when we're in that head-over-heels state, it's awfully easy to overlook the parts of ourselves that might not be so compatible.

It sure felt great, though. When it worked, while it worked, it *really* worked.

I'll never forget our New Year's Eve. It was my first New Year's as a fit and healthy man, and I decided to do something really special. I made plans to take Sarah to a lavish, black-tie gala at a fancy hotel in San Francisco, and since I knew I was never, ever going to put on weight again, I decided to buy a tuxedo. Not to rent one. To *buy* one.

In my mind, there was only one place to go to do that.

I walked into the Nordstrom in Palo Alto feeling down-right triumphant. This was my redemption. Not only did I look good, and feel good, but I could afford this: since I'd hit my goal weight and started running, and become a more social person, my career had gone through the roof. I carried myself with confidence. I radiated a passion for life, and that passion carried over into every part of my life, including my job. Being an appliance salesman still wasn't the career I dreamed about as a kid, but it became so much more fun and enjoyable once I felt better in my body—and once I felt better about *me*.

So I stepped into the tuxedo section at Nordstrom, ready for redemption, looking like a well-heeled man on a mission. A sales associate approached me within seconds. Before I knew it, I was trying on tuxes with a team of associates whirling around me, suggesting different styles and cuts and fabrics. I settled on a classic Burberry in black, and I stood on a step stool in front of a three-sided mirror, looking at myself in triplicate while the on-site tailor marked my measurements with pins and chalk.

They offered me a real, tie-it-yourself bow tie, and cuff links, and suspenders, and I bought those, too. I wanted to look sharp. The last time I had worn a tux was for my high school junior prom, which I went to with my high school sweetheart, Jaye. I wore a powder blue ruffled shirt back then. Needless to say, styles had changed. I purchased a crisp white tuxedo shirt, and when I asked about a cummer-bund, the salesperson advised me that they'd gone out of style years ago and that I should go with suspenders instead.

They asked if I needed shoes, and I said, "Of course!"

And the staff brought shoes to me rather than making me walk all the way over to the shoe department. The pair I liked best was $600. The tuxedo was $1,200 on sale. With all of the accoutrements, I dropped more than two grand in that one visit—but I left feeling like a million bucks.

Sarah and I enjoyed a magical, romantic New Year's evening that neither of us would ever forget.

That relationship and those months spent together filled me with happiness like I'd rarely known. And being with Sarah served as a bridge to more friendships than I'd made in the entire second half of my life—in part because our plan to throw a vegan dinner party quickly expanded itself into a wildly successful series of local social events.

The first dinner was held at my condo. It wound up being just Sarah and a couple of other friends for a low-key night in. But as Sarah and those other friends talked about the food I prepared, other members of our runners group started asking if they could join in. By the third dinner, I wound up hosting ten people in my condo and cooking for all of them myself like a gourmet chef in my formerly unused kitchen.

Peety loved it. He was absolutely thrilled to see so many people in our home. He greeted every new person at the door, then led them toward the balcony. He seemed to walk around to each one of them with a wag of the tail and a happy look on his face, eliciting more than his fair share of pets and hugs from everyone he could.

Vicki brought her young son along on that night. She didn't have a sitter, and at first he didn't want to come along to a "boring" dinner full of adults. But when she told him about Peety, he agreed. I had never seen Peety interact with a child before. I was a little nervous about it ahead of their arrival. After all, Casaundra had warned me that I should be careful with him around children, and she specifically picked me as a match for Peety because I didn't have any kids.

All of my worry melted away the moment Vicki's son walked through the door. Mason saw my hardwood floor and took his shoes off and went running down the hall, sliding in his socks, and Peety ran right along with him, barking at the excitement of his newfound friend. I heard some growling a few minutes later and poked my head out of the kitchen to make sure everything was OK, and Mason was down on the floor, wrestling with Peety and rolling around. Peety was in heaven!

I remember thinking, *Wow. OK. Maybe he was only "bad" with children the way I was "bad" with women. Maybe he was just a cranky old guy because of his health. Maybe it was just because he was in pain and felt alone and rejected all the time.*

I also had this glimmer of a vision that maybe Peety would like to find himself in a home full of kids someday, in a family, where there was more than one person to love besides me, his dear old dad. He clearly had plenty of love to give.

I suppose that meant I was starting to feel a glimmer of hope for a family myself.

Sarah and I settled on a Spanish theme for that first big party. We served organic, fruity sangria during cocktail hour. We decorated my apartment with streamers and twinkly lights to accentuate the already-Spanish theme of my decorating scheme. I came up with some fun "tapas" appetizers for everyone to nibble on while I put the finishing touches on my signature vegan paella. And when I walked out into the living room to announce that dinner was ready, I noticed everyone in the room was basically standing over in one corner.

"Why are you all over there?" I asked. Everyone looked around and laughed.

"Peety pushed me over here," Vicki said.

"Me, too!" Sarah echoed.

"Yeah, me, too!" everyone else agreed.

Peety had apparently herded all of them together!

"Peety!" I said. "Relax, dude. I know you're a herding dog, but this is a party. There's no need to work the living room, son."

Everyone in the group got a kick out of it—and everyone really seemed to enjoy the dinner.

"I thought it would be fun to hang out," Vicki said after the last course, "but I had no idea vegan food could be this good. I really expected something, I dunno...bland."

Everyone laughed at that, and more than one of the new guests said, "Yeah, me, too."

"Well, look, I'm happy to share recipes and show any of you how to make this stuff. Just call me," I said.

"Heck, I'm gonna hire you to come cook for me!" Vicki said, holding her glass high in the air.

"Cheers to that!" Sarah responded.

We all toasted, and I decided to one-up her. "Tell you what, Vicki. You host next time. I'll do the cooking for free, but we'll do it as a fund-raiser for Humane Society Silicon Valley, in Peety's name."

"Done!" Vicki said.

"Can Peety come over, too?" her son asked.

"Of course!" I said.

Mason ran to Peety's side and said, "You're coming to my house, boy! Won't that be fun?"

Next thing I knew, Vicki and Sarah had the whole thing planned out, and a few weeks later we turned Vicki's kitchen into a Moroccan oasis. We cooked the meal together so everyone could learn some new techniques, and the food was out of this world. I spent days beforehand discovering new spices. I stopped by some Moroccan restaurants and asked their chefs for some pointers. We spun all of that research into a plant-based version of a "chicken tagine" (made with tofu), and a whole menu full of deliciousness that filled everyone's senses with an array of surprising new scents and flavors.

They all wanted more. So we planned more events. We did a Thai theme, and a Chinese theme, and a Vietnamese theme, and circled back to the Spanish theme more than once. As others learned to cook new dishes, they hosted— either with my help or without—serving foods as simple as portobello mushroom "burgers" that hadn't even occurred to me to make myself. We wound up with people on waiting lists trying to get in to these events. We wound up raising money for a few great causes because of it, and the cama- raderie carried into phone calls and e-mails and text mes- sages and Facebook connections that stay with me to this day. Along the way, there were more and more doggie play dates to be had, and date nights with Sarah, and more and more of us got into running together, too.

During those dinners, so many people began asking me questions about how and why the whole-food, plant-based diet worked for me that I decided I wanted to offer them more than my own personal, anecdotal stories in response. So I enrolled in a series of science and medical courses at a local community college. I got hooked and wound up completing the entire first-year course requirements for med school in my spare time, just to try to get to the bottom of why Dr. Preeti's plan had worked so well for me, and to try to understand why we have such a large obesity problem in this country. (Pun intended.) I took anatomy, physiology, chemistry, organic chemistry, biology, nutrition science, and even physics and psychology.

I used my research skills as a former attorney for those classes. When you hear about new nutrition studies on the news, it's impossible to tell whether the information has been properly vetted, or whether it's just hype or marketing. So whenever I did research, I looked at the studies carefully to see who funded them, how they were performed, and if they were biased. I weighed the evidence and compared conflicting results. I dug into medical journals. I learned about the cellular processing of nutrients in food. I learned about our bone structure and every muscle in the human body. Through all of that training, I learned how to really read food labels and to understand the meaning of every word on every package in the grocery store. But there was something else I discovered on a broader scale, and to this day I cannot understand why this information isn't widely known.

What experts have concluded in peer-reviewed studies is this: if every person in America transitioned to a whole-food, plant-based diet and engaged in a lifestyle with the sort of physical activity that their grandparents practiced, we could save up to a trillion dollars a year in health care costs. The side effect of that is that 75 percent or more of all chronic disease would be alleviated. Seventy-five percent! The modern epidemic of heart attacks, strokes, and most cancers would be greatly reduced. Type 2 diabetes would be all but eliminated. This isn't my opinion. This is now generally accepted scientific knowledge, which for some reason hasn't yet filtered into the popular view of the world. The medical profession is still not advocating for significant changes in diet. They're still prescribing pills because of the economics of the system. In modern medical practice, most doctors only have about five minutes to spend with each patient. That's only enough time to hear a complaint and prescribe a medication to alleviate the complaint. Nothing more.

I wanted to scream to every doctor in America: "Why aren't we prescribing nutrition instead?!"

The more I learned, the more I wanted to find a way to share what I'd learned with others. I thought about completing my coursework to become a registered dietician, but I couldn't see myself starting a new profession from scratch at my age. So I didn't do it. I thought about it, though, and I took every prerequisite class seriously.

The more I learned about health and the more I embraced the empowerment of leading a healthy lifestyle, the more passionate I grew about running. People talk about a runner's high, and it definitely exists. All of those endorphins get pumping while you run, and it made me feel incredible. I never would have believed that had I not experienced it for myself. Before long, I found myself sleeping for no more than seven hours every night, and I woke up every day actually craving a good run, the way I used to crave pizza and Egg McMuffins.

Along with Sarah and Vicki, and wholly against my better judgment, I entered myself into a race that spring. It wasn't a marathon. It wasn't even a half marathon. I knew I could cover the distance. But the idea of pushing myself to try to win a race set off every insecurity I had. In my mind, no matter how I looked in the mirror I still saw myself as Pudge—the fat kid who couldn't run the bases and wasn't able to get over a three-foot fence.

Lo and behold, I finished that race with a respectable time. My endorphins were pumping more than ever. It actually felt kind of incredible to push myself. I liked the way it felt to set a goal and set a pace, so I could get to the finish line as quickly as possible without wearing myself out along the way. And I loved the unbelievable high of achieving that goal. I loved the camaraderie of celebrating with everyone at the finish line, while feeling an individual pride over my body's still-unexpected and unbelievably surprising capabilities.

Somewhere along the way in those six months, though, Sarah and I started to drift apart. It seemed as if she wasn't happy unless she was planning the next event. We began fighting over stupid little meaningless things, and when I had to miss one of her events for a business trip, she treated it as a personal affront. In many ways, it just seemed to me that Sarah and I weren't all that compatible beyond the bedroom and the running trail. We wound up getting in a fight one night on a sailboat, surrounded by a bunch of our mutual runner friends. I don't even remember what started it, but we'd both had a little too much to drink, and everything just came bubbling to the surface. It was awful. Sarah unfriended and even blocked me on Facebook. She didn't want to be around me anymore. She cut me out of her life completely, which meant that I had to go find another runners group to join.

That reaction was devastating, and for a few days, I felt as alone as I'd ever felt.

I remained friends with most of the other members of that runners group, though. They reached out to me, and that felt good. I remain friends with most of them to this day.

Peety comforted me in that loss the way he comforted me in everything. I couldn't lock myself in my condo and not go outside. I had to go outside to walk him. No matter what. And that got me moving. And then we ate together. And even when I didn't shower for two days, he looked up at me, always, like I was the greatest guy in the world.

Finally, one evening, I had a glass of bourbon with Peety next to me and blared George Jones's "He Stopped Loving Her Today" on the stereo. I'm not sure Peety understood the lyrics, but he howled out of tune with the song a bit, and after that I was OK.

Faster than I ever would have imagined possible, I came to grips with the fact that my relationship with Sarah may have just been a stepping-stone to the rest of my life. And even though I was heartbroken, I was grateful for it. For one thing, I was happy to know that I had a heart to break! But I was also thankful for everything Sarah had given to me.

Sarah was someone who brought people together. She made connections. I admired her for that, and I wanted to emulate her passion for that in my own life.

She was the woman who brought me back. To experience a relationship with another person, especially someone who I previously may have considered unattainably attractive, gave me a newfound confidence. A confidence that I felt pretty sure would never, ever fade away.

Within a week of the breakup I connected with another running group, and I went ahead and entered myself in an upcoming race, just so I would have something to look forward to. I decided I needed to dive back into life with everything I had, and I did.

As my passion for running grew, and my passion for plant-based eating grew, so did my passion for animals. As I told my new friends on numerous occasions, Peety was the reason I became a new person. He was my conduit to the world, my greatest supporter, my true companion, the one who loved me unconditionally and brought me continuous joy. The more I thought about what he had done for me, the more I wanted to do whatever I could to see that animals like Peety were protected—that they were rescued, and cared for, and given the resources and opportunities necessary to find their way into people's lives.

I sometimes looked around at the grumpy faces at the airport and the appliance stores I visited and wondered how much nicer the world would be if everybody had a dog.

Before all of this began, I wasn't an animal-rights type of guy. Greenpeace and PETA and those sappy, Sarah

McLachlan–themed "save a dog" commercials for the ASPCA never touched my heart. Now? All of it touched my heart. I began to think of animals as "the least among us." The thought of Peety or any living creature like him being caged up or abused or cut up for food was just too much to bear.

I kept asking myself, "Why?" Why was any of it necessary? God gave us a bounty of more than twenty thousand edible plants on this planet, in endlessly renewable quantities, offering all of the nutrition and nourishment we could ever want or need, and those food sources could be cooked into endless possibilities of flavors and textures suitable to every palate—even a palate as vegetable-opposed as mine! Almost all of those foods are easy to grow without any negative impact on the environment, or our bodies, and without destroying animals in the process of producing *or* consuming them. So why do we continue to ignore all of that and choose something else entirely?

I won't go into every detail here. The stats are available and well documented to anyone who opens their eyes to them. Anyone who wants to know more can do what I did: watch the documentaries *Forks over Knives*, *Cowspiracy*, and *What the Health*. (You can find them on Netflix.) But with all of the science and everything we now know about how destructive the commercialized farming of animals is to the planet, and how awful it is for the animals themselves, and how harmful animal products are to our bodies—there are major studies showing that meat and dairy carry similar carcinogenic risks to cigarettes—why do we find it necessary to perpetuate these broken ways of living?

Once I turned that corner, once I opened my eyes, I found support for my new way of thinking seemingly everywhere I turned, including in the Bible right there at my bedside.

It seemed increasingly clear to me that from the beginning, God wanted our source of food to be the plants and trees all around us:

> *Then God said, "Look! I have given you every*
> *seed-bearing plant throughout the earth and*
> *all the fruit trees for your food."*
> —Genesis 1:29 (NLT)

One day, I saw a Facebook ad for a PETA Pack run to be held at the Presidio in San Francisco, and I decided I wanted to show my support to that organization by joining. I e-mailed the organizer, a woman named Michelle, and offered not only to run, but also to help her in any way I could. I was so enthusiastic and passionate about finding a direct intersection of animal rights and running, I probably came off a little over-the-top to her. We met at an organizing event and talked for what seemed like hours. She was clearly passionate about these issues, too, and she seemed to enjoy my perspective on the importance of a whole-food, plant-based diet. In fact, she was so enthusiastic about what I had to say that she invited me to speak at an upcoming PETA event.

Without even asking, my hopes of finding an outlet to share all of my newfound knowledge found *me*.

A few weeks later, I stood up in front of a large audience in a conference room, and I began my first-ever PowerPoint presentation aimed at a crowd of animal lovers and activists. After Michelle introduced me, and the audience had a chance to see me and get to know me for a moment, in my currently in-shape body, and as a runner who had participated in their fund-raising program, I turned the projector on and showed them a photo of me when I weighed in at 340 pounds.

The audience audibly gasped.

From that point forward, they were hooked. And this is what I told them:

"What we eat is a function of physical need, what we prefer, what we have available, and what we believe." They listened intently.

"Let's begin by defining some basic terms," I said. "Carnivores eat other animals exclusively, but not plants. Omnivores are people or animals that eat some plants and some animals. People on the 'paleo' diet believe they are eating a similar diet to cavemen. Pescatarians are people who only eat fish and plants. Vegetarians eat dairy products, eggs, and plants. Vegans only eat plant foods. But in this talk, I will refer to myself as someone who follows a whole-food, plant-based diet, rather than as someone who is on a vegan diet. Why? Because I only eat healthy vegan food rather than vegan junk food. So I strive to only eat foods prepared from whole plants, with no added oil or sugar, rather than processed foods that include added oil, sugar, and other additives."

I asked, "Why would anyone only eat plants, and not meat, fish, chicken, eggs, or dairy?" I paused, then continued. "For three main reasons: for reasons related to health, ethics involving animal exploitation, and for environmental reasons.

"Can everyone live well just by eating plants? Yes. According to the official position of the American Dietetic Association, well-planned vegetarian and vegan diets are healthful for individuals during all stages of the life cycle, including pregnancy, lactation, infancy, childhood, and adolescence, and for athletes. But is eating just plants healthier than an omnivore diet? Again, the answer is yes. But rather than just give my opinion based on my own experience, let's discuss the facts.

"The evidence that a whole-food, plant-based diet is superior to an omnivore diet is as clear as the evidence that you can develop lung cancer from smoking cigarettes, and that greenhouse gases produced by human activity are affecting our environment. There are some who may deny these facts, but they are generally accepted by the great majority of the credible scientific and medical community. Legions of written accounts with numerous credible witnesses who have spent their lives studying and proving these facts can attest to their accuracy. And the facts are these: seventy percent of Americans are now either obese or overweight." I showed them a slide with the research to back up that claim, citing a report by the Centers for Disease Control. In fact, all of the studies I used to support my case were published in mainstream journals. These weren't from extremist or activist websites. As I mentioned, this isn't fringe science. It's generally accepted science.

"We are doing something wrong, people, and we are headed even farther in the wrong direction. Meat and cheese consumption has similar mortality risks to smoking," I told them, citing a study published by the National Institutes of Health.

"Right now, the majority of non-vegans need statins to reduce their cholesterol to healthy levels," I added, citing a report from the *American Heart Journal*. "Studies show that if you don't consume animal products or added oils, your cholesterol will most likely remain at healthy levels, and you are unlikely to experience sudden death from a heart attack.

"But consumption of animal products is responsible for much more than just heart attacks. In fact, over seventy-five percent of chronic disease—type 2 diabetes, heart attack, stroke, and cancer—can be eliminated with a plant-based diet," I said, again citing mainstream research that studied large populations over long periods of time. "So if these facts are true, why isn't everyone on a whole-food, plant-based diet?" I spoke about my five-minute doctor visits and how the medical establishment is programmed to treat symptoms rather than underlying causes. "Think of the difference like this: When you turn on a water spigot, water runs out onto the floor. The symptom is water running out onto the floor. If you try to cure the problem by mopping up the water, you will never stop mopping. If instead, you turn off the spigot, you have cured the underlying problem. So doctors give most patients drugs instead of explaining the plant-based option because they don't have time to explain the benefits and necessity of a plant-based diet. They also assume their patients won't follow nutritional advice." I had evidence to back up that claim, too, taken directly from *The American Journal of Cardiology*.

"Another reason: just follow the money. There is no money in dead people. There is no money in healthy people, either—they have nothing to cure. All of the money is in sick people. Our entire health care industry, medical insurance industry, and animal agricultural industry benefit from people overeating unhealthy foods, because that maximizes their cash flows and profits."

The audience lapped it up. When I finished, a reception line formed and I stood there for over an hour shaking people's hands, hearing their stories, and answering their questions. That one talk would lead to me being asked to do presentations at obesity groups, recovery groups, AA meetings, church meetings, and more.

I also made an impact on a personal level. At the end of the night, a particularly cute redhead with a white poodle stuck around to flirt with me. She asked me if I'd like to go for a drink. And I said, "Sure."

# chapter 17

# At Your Service

One thing was clear: women had become more assertive during my fifteen-year hibernation.

Back when I first started walking Peety at Emma Prusch Farm Park, I dreamed that one day, one of those women out walking her own dog might notice me and find me attractive. What soon became clear is that this formerly innocent-looking park full of chickens was actually a bit of a pick-up scene. With Peety as my wingman, the conversations always began with him, and now that I was single again and carrying myself with confidence, I found that I didn't even have to get up the nerve to ask these women for coffee. Nine times out of ten, *they* were the ones asking *me*.

It happened at speaking engagements, running meet-ups, and road races, too. I entered a two-year phase of casual dating that was far more fun than I ever imagined a fifty-something-year-old man could have. Feeling attractive made me feel young. Actually, I felt better than young. Even when I was dating in my twenties, I never felt so good. For the first time in my life I had full confidence in myself, and in my body.

Until my body failed me.

Over the course of 2011 and 2012, I started running almost every day, and I gradually stepped my races up from 5Ks to half marathons to full marathons over the course of a single year. Not only was each jump in distance a major accomplishment for me, but I kept improving my times as well. Running became exactly what Dr. Preeti had hoped I'd find in an exercise routine: something I enjoyed, and something that could become a lifelong passion.

By the fall of 2012, I think it's fair to say that I had become an athlete. That nagging, internal feeling that I was nothing more than a grown-up Pudge completely vanished. When I thought about that long-ago kid, and even the man I was two years earlier, he felt like someone else; like an old acquaintance, a grammar school friend, or a former colleague you got along with just fine but who isn't a part of your life anymore, and knowing you'll never see him again doesn't make you the least bit sad.

Feeling the authority of my muscles, tuning in to the sound of my own breath, experiencing the commanding heartbeat in my chest as I ran with the sun on my face and the wind at my back, I felt strong. I felt powerful. At times I felt almost invincible.

Then on October 28, 2012, I woke up in a hospital bed with no memory of what had happened or how I got there. The ER doctor informed me that I'd suffered a seizure. I'd blacked out on mile 21 of the Morgan Hill Marathon.

It was the only race I'd ever run with a result marked "DNF"—Did Not Finish.

The medical team ran a series of tests. They ruled out a stroke or a heart attack, but the results of the tests were otherwise inconclusive. They suggested I'd simply pushed myself too hard on the run and my body had shut itself down. They fed me some overpriced aspirin, told me to get some rest, and, after a night of observation in the hospital, sent me home.

What I didn't tell the ER doc is that I was pretty sure I knew what caused my blackout—and dehydration or my passion for running was not to blame.

When people pass out or die during a run, so many people, including doctors, tend to blame the act of running for what happened. Every day, people use stories of famous runners who dropped dead in their running shoes as an excuse not to run themselves. But running itself is almost never the cause. The cause is almost always some underlying problem—a heart condition, or in my case, a brain injury.

It's not something I liked to talk about. The symptoms hadn't shown up in so many years, I'd all but forgotten it happened. But during my time in the army, I suffered a traumatic brain injury during a training exercise. I wound up in the infirmary for weeks, and for a few years afterward I suffered occasional blackouts and seizures with no warning. They were scary. I worried about what might happen if one hit while I was painting high up on a water tower, or worse, if I was driving. But more often than not, they happened in the comfort of my own apartment, and there never seemed to be any lasting effects. I always recovered with ease as soon as the spell was over, and eventually the spells stopped. I hadn't had an incident in so long, I truly assumed that my old injury had healed itself.

In the wake of that new blackout, I went to see a brain specialist, and after running some tests he confirmed my suspicion: my TBI was the only reasonable explanation for what had happened to me at mile 21.

I talked with my therapist about it, too, and told her that I thought it was a fluke.

"I'm not too worried about it happening again," I said.

I was lying. I was very worried. I was terrified that this brain injury could put an end to my new life. *What if the blackouts start happening frequently again? What if it affects my work? What if the Department of Motor Vehicles finds out and takes my driver's license? What if the stress of worrying about it causes me to stop running? What if I start gaining weight?*

My therapist saw through my bravado right away. She knew me pretty well by that point, and she insisted that we do something about it.

A year or so earlier I had inquired about whether I might be able to get Peety some sort of certification as a service dog so I could bring him with me wherever I went. It was a naive question, and after reviewing my case, my therapist eventually gave me a flat "no."

First of all, it's not the dog that gets "certified" for such a thing. Under the ADA, a person with a disability is entitled to travel with and be accompanied by a dog trained to assist the person with his or her disability. Peety certainly brought me a lot of comfort. He was the reason I didn't lose my way when I felt like I couldn't go on. But since I didn't have a physical disability, and I didn't suffer from clinical depression or another psychological condition, my therapist could not prescribe a service dog for me—and I completely understood the law and facts relating to her decision. Imagine the chaos in the world if anyone who simply wanted the comfort of a dog's companionship was able to bring untrained dogs onto airplanes and into schools and restaurants. We'd have dogs and other pets climbing everywhere and disrupting the basic functions of society. It just wouldn't work. The ADA standards are specific for a reason.

But revealing my TBI changed everything.

"Even if you weren't a dog lover already, knowing you have a brain injury that can cause you to have seizures or lose consciousness, I would recommend that you obtain a service dog, one that is trained to alert others and get you help if you suffer a blackout."

"Can't I just get one of those medic-alert devices? You know, 'I've fallen and I can't get up!'?"

"Those devices generally have to be triggered by pushing a button, so they wouldn't do much for you if you're unconscious," she said.

"I was just kidding."

"Well I'm not. This is potentially a very dangerous condition, Eric. I'm not sure if your dog—"

"Peety," I said.

"That's right, Peety. I'm not sure if Peety can be trained for this. Perhaps he's up to the task, I don't know. But if not, I recommend that you acquire another dog, a trained service dog, to be with you for your own safety. In fact, I'm going to put you in touch with a couple of organizations that work with service animals so you can get the process started."

And just like that, my old injury turned into an unexpected gift.

Of course Peety was up to the task. *He's a herder. He's a working dog by nature*, I thought. *Heck, he's smarter than many people I know!* We went through the training together and he learned everything like a pro. First he had to solidify the regimen of basic commands—sit, stay, down, etc.—which we did through a system of rewards. Practicing the word "sit" while I pressed on his back with one hand and held a treat in my other hand only took three or four times before Peety fully recognized that "sit" and his bottom being on the ground led to a tasty mouthful of deliciousness. "Heel" was a tougher one, since he was used to walking out in front of me, but he caught onto that pretty quickly, too. So much of my bonding with Peety was over food, and delicious all-natural treats served as quite the motivator.

The last part of the training called for Peety to bark and go get help should I black out and hit the ground, and he was a natural. The fact is, a dog that loves you tends to freak out naturally if you hit the floor. So training him to act like Lassie, to bark and run to seek the help of another human if I had another episode, was almost as easy as teaching him to sit.

There is no official certification for service dogs in the United States. There are no tags or papers or special IDs. Vests are not required, and they're only used by those who choose to have the world know instantly that their dogs are on the clock. And for all of those reasons there are people out there who sometimes try to pass their dogs off as service dogs just to get them onto planes and into public places. I've read about all sorts of cases where people made up fake IDs and even dressed their dogs in fake vests just to avoid a pet deposit or circumvent a "no pets allowed" policy that they didn't agree with. But doing this is unethical and disrespectful to people with disabilities and the animals trained to help them. The laws about faking a service dog are strict, too. False claims can be punishable with fines, jail time, and the dogs can even be taken away from their owners. Since there's a lot of controversy and confusion around these issues, I made up my mind to learn all I could and to try to educate people about the process, and the law, whenever they asked. And wherever Peety went with me, people asked.

Mostly, though, I just felt blessed. The idea that Peety could help me if I blacked out was astonishing to me. He had already given me so much, and yet I gained a whole new level of appreciation for him during our training. If I had any doubts that this dog was sent from heaven, this twist of fate certainly put those doubts to rest.

Knowing that I had him as an added layer of protection in my life gave me the confidence to know that I was going to be OK. If I had another blackout, Peety would be there, watching over me and protecting me.

I didn't think that bringing Peety on planes would be a great idea, so I never attempted it with him. I figured I would be surrounded by people at airports and business meetings anyway, and they could call for help if something happened. And I didn't worry too much about something happening in the confines of a hotel room.

Peety also couldn't come running with me. I tried it on a few occasions and he just wasn't into it. So during runs, I would be vulnerable. But that's why I ran with friends, in groups, always in a social environment.

I never ran alone. And with Peety, I never walked alone.

Of course, there was an added bonus to being prescribed a service dog: I now had permission to take Peety anywhere we wanted to go. So we went.

As soon as I had a day off we made our way back into San Francisco. I walked up to the ticket booth near Pier 39 and asked for a ticket to tour Alcatraz.

"There are no dogs allowed on our boats, sir," the young lady behind the counter told me.

"He's a service dog," I said.

"What service?" she asked.

She had every right to ask that question. In fact, according to the U.S. Department of Justice, there are two questions that federal law allows a business to ask in response to a service dog claim. One: Is this a service dog required because of disability? And two: What is the dog trained to do to mitigate the disability?

The first question is sort of redundant. The answer is, "Yes, this is a service dog." But then, if a business asks what the dog is specifically trained to do to assist me with my disability, I am required to answer with information about the specific defined task. It cannot be a claim of general comfort.

So I answered, and she sold me my ticket.

Peety hopped on board his very first boat like a seasoned sailor. He no longer suffered the hesitations he had when we first met, when he struggled to get into my car and balked at stepping into an elevator. He had confidence now. He walked easily with the sway of the waves, and he leaned into the rail and looked out at the water and seagulls as we took off toward the crumbling old prison on the giant rock in the middle of the bay.

Peety was patient and quiet during the tour. I was really impressed with what a good boy he was. Other people on the boat and inside the prison were surprised to see a dog and asked all about him, then asked if they could pet him. I said, "Sure." Many service dogs should not be distracted, and they wear marked vests to indicate that they should not be touched. But this was not the case with Peety, and he loved the extra attention from strangers.

The only doggie infraction Peety made during our excursion was when they showed us Al Capone's cell: Cell 133 on B-Block. For some reason, in that particularly charged and some say "haunted" location, Peety felt the need to mark his territory. He lifted his leg and peed on Al Capone's cell bars!

I was glad the tour guide wasn't looking. The last thing we wanted to do was get in trouble. It was somehow fitting that Peety left his mark on that landmark, though. I couldn't help but wonder how many dogs had ever been to Alcatraz. It was just such a gift to have him along, as my savior, as my companion and friend, while we both got a chance to do a little sightseeing. He deserved to see those sights, I thought. I wanted him to see the world. He'd been caged up and tied down for far too long.

Come to think of it, so had I.

I made a vow to take Peety on daytrips and sightseeing adventures every chance I could. He was my special dog, and from that day forward I wanted him to go where most dogs couldn't. In the coming months, we'd take all sorts of little journeys around the Bay Area. I took him to swim in the ocean for the first time, and laughed as he sprinted through the sand, the same way he'd always sprinted to the duck pond at Penitencia Creek Park. I took him for a ride on a miniature train, where he sat in a seat in a little train car and went around and around like all of the other little boys and girls. I took him to restaurants—although it turns out he was a little rambunctious for that setting, which made me quickly limit our dining excursions to outdoor seating areas. The last thing I wanted to do was disturb other people who were out eating and having a good time. The point of our travels together was not to cause problems.

In fact, I was surprised at how accommodating most people were when I told them Peety was a service dog. It was like suddenly the walls came down and they looked at him as something more than a pet or a nuisance. They looked at him with respect. Most people seemed proud to let the two of us into their establishment, be it a hotel, a restaurant, a mom-and-pop shop, a bank, or an auto repair shop.

Peety's constant companionship added an interesting element to my dating life, too. It was unusual and exciting for my dates to walk into a restaurant with a dog, and they were blown away that Peety would just lie on the ground, content to be with me, no matter the setting. It gave us something to talk about, too, and laugh about, and it helped some of the women I dated to open up about their own experiences with pets and animals through the years. They told stories about horses, or their beloved cats and dogs that always knew when they were sick as a child, and who would always comfort them in times of need. I even heard stories about bunnies with big personalities. Who knew bunnies had personalities?

I also came to trust Peety's judgment implicitly. If he warmed up to somebody, chances are I would warm up to them, too. If he didn't warm up to somebody, I could tell that we probably weren't compatible. And if he didn't like someone at all, I immediately steered clear. One of my friends insisted that Peety was an "evil detector." It was so strange how during our walks he would ignore most people, and then every once in a while he would growl at a complete stranger. It's almost as if he could see their hearts, or their souls, or their auras, or something.

Whatever it was he saw, I trusted it.

The thing about the dating scene is that it grows old pretty quickly. After a couple years of bouncing around, I fell into the same place I had in my twenties. I grew tired of the games and the constant effort it takes to get to know somebody new, only to have it end quickly and then be forced to start the process all over again. I wanted something more stable. I wanted something deeper. And those brief fleeting thoughts about how much Peety might like to be a part of a family someday seemed to keep coming back.

It was right around this time that I stopped dating women who didn't share my values. My respect for animals and the choices I'd made about food were both absolutely essential ingredients of my personal happiness, and I found it difficult to bond with and experience intimacy with people who didn't share these same values. I accepted that other people had different views, and I wasn't so strict that I couldn't sit at a table with people who ate meat. But the idea of having a deep relationship with a woman whose views weren't in line with mine just didn't seem possible.

Since it can be uncomfortable to ask someone about their diet before you even ask them to dinner, I decided the best way to meet other single people with the same values as me would be to join a vegan singles meet-up group. (Yes, there are vegan-singles meet-up groups in California. They exist in lots of other places now, too.)

Turns out it was a very good move.

## chapter 18

# Sweet Melissa

When Melissa walked into the restaurant, she caught my eye before we spoke a word to each other. She was younger. Maybe much younger. And the effervescent energy of her personality seemed to light up the entire room.

I was early that night, the first to arrive at the meet-up. I knew the restaurant, and since it was small, crowded, and extremely loud, I thought it was best to leave Peety at home. Melissa arrived maybe a minute after I got there. She introduced herself and we had a chance to talk for a few minutes one-on-one. It turned out she had organized this group herself because she, too, had given up on dating those who didn't share her views on food, animals, and the environment. The only problem, she said, was she'd held a bunch of these meet-ups and still hadn't met any guys she was interested in. "Most of the guys who come to these meet-ups are tech guys who recently came here from India and were raised on a vegetarian diet. They're really nice guys, but there are huge cultural differences between us and we never seem to have much in common. Most of them aren't even vegan! The only other guys who show up are these really over-the-top hippie-activist types, which, you know, isn't *me*," she said.

Melissa came off like a driven young professional. Her clothes were conservative. Her hair wasn't streaked with any funky colors or dreadlocks.

"Yeah. I hear you. A lot of vegans in the Bay Area seem to fall into the hippie category—"

"Don't they? Why is that?" she said. We both laughed. "I don't know, I work a regular job, I'm in sales—"

"Me, too," I said.

"Really? That's cool. I've been vegetarian since I was eight, and went vegan when I was ten, so it's who I am. I don't eat or wear any animal products, period. I'm clearly more of a junk food vegan, I mean, *look at me*," she said. "But it's important to me. I need it to be important to anyone I want to even think about having a relationship with. So that's why I started this group, to give it a shot, you know?"

I hadn't even noticed that she was overweight until she made that "look at me" comment. All I saw was a bright shining smile and eyes filled with hope on a pretty, five-foot-five-inch frame.

A couple of other guys joined us at that point. They walked over and introduced themselves and said they both worked in the tech industry, and had both moved to Silicon Valley from India recently to pursue their careers. Melissa gave me a look, like, "See what I mean?"

Another woman who looked to be in her thirties soon

joined us, and another young man of Vietnamese descent. When we all sat down for dinner, Melissa sat right next to me. I took that as a good sign.

She asked me how long ago I had stopped eating animal products, and I told her my whole story. I asked her to tell me more about herself, and she noted that nearly her entire family was vegetarian. It started with her mom, and then Melissa jumped on board because she was such an animal lover, and eventually her four siblings turned to plant-based diets themselves. The only one who didn't was her dad.

She was a heavyset kid, she said, just like I'd been, but switching to a vegan diet at age ten helped her slim down through most of her school years. As time went on, she started eating chips and all sorts of prepackaged vegan "junk food," filled with flavor but low on nutrition. I noticed for dinner that night she ordered a vegan "sweet-and-sour shrimp" dish—a dish filled with tofu covered with a syrupy glaze and few vegetables. She seemed fascinated by the fact that I'd lost so much weight on a plant-based diet, and she wanted to know how. Especially since she'd tried everything under the sun to lose weight herself, from Weight Watchers and other commercial diet plans, to taking Ephedra, back when those diet pills were still legal.

It struck me how similar her weight-gain story was to mine. She hit a point in time when her metabolism changed, and the weight just kept adding up, a little bit more after every attempt she made to lose weight with a diet.

"I just couldn't stick with anything," she said. "All of the food was boring and bland, and I always felt underfed. I've been around the two-hundred-pound mark for about eight years now, and it's just awful. I have two boys who are filled with energy, and I get home after work and feel like a slug. Every day. I never go clothes shopping. I hate it. Other women love clothes shopping and talk about it like it's their favorite sport, and I just can't stand it. Nothing fits. It's just torturous."

"I get it. I completely get it," I said.

"I'm sorry. I shouldn't be sitting here complaining. Life is good, right? We're here! We're eating good food. I had no idea I'd meet someone like you tonight. I mean, life is good, *right*?"

I smiled. "Life is great," I said.

As we walked out of the restaurant, I asked Melissa if she was on Facebook. She said she was. She gave me her e-mail address and asked me to look her up. I sent her a friend request that night, and she accepted it within minutes.

Melissa put together another meet-up event the following weekend, and nearly the same group of people showed up, plus one or two others. We sat next to each other again, and the whole group seemed to fade into the background. She told me some funny stories about her boys, Joey and Mike, and I told her some funny stories about Peety.

At some point I mentioned the dinner parties I'd thrown at my condo.

"Oh, my gosh! Could we do one of these at your place sometime? Would you cook for us? I mean, I've never heard anyone describe food the way you describe food, let alone *vegan* food. I mean, it's kind of exciting to think about!"

"Yeah," I said. "Sure. Maybe six or eight people. I could make my paella."

"That sounds awesome! All right. I'll put it together," she said. "And maybe I can come be your sous chef."

"That would be awesome," I said.

"There's just one problem. I can't cook."

"Then you'll have to come extra early so I can teach you," I said.

She smiled and looked into my eyes, and I got butterflies in my stomach. I hoped to God that she felt it, too.

"Well, then," she said. "That sounds even better."

Her leg brushed against mine, and I felt that tingle—that sensation when every cell in your body wants to make that connection go further. I felt a little flush and suddenly embarrassed. I broke eye contact and looked down at the table.

"You know, I'm probably old enough to be your grandfather," I said.

"What?! How old do you think I am?" she said with a laugh. "I'm not *that* young."

"How young is not young?"

"I'm twenty-eight," she said. "Wait, how old are *you*?"

"I'm not telling," I said.

"Come on!"

"Guess."

"I'm guessing like forty-three," she said.

"Let's just go with that for now, OK?"

"Oh, my God! How old *are* you?"

"Forty-three sounds good. You're only as old as you think you are, right?"

"All right, mister. I'll let it slide for now, but I'm gonna get it out of you sooner or later."

"When the time is right, I'll tell you," I said.

"Deal."

Melissa and I started talking on the phone and sending Facebook messages to each other, and the act of planning our paella dinner came together as smoothly as any dinner party I'd ever organized with Sarah. That scared me a little. I hoped I wasn't repeating myself. I really liked Melissa. Something about her energy and her spirit got me excited. Not just physically excited, but excited for *life*. I felt like I wanted to show off for her, and teach her, and share things with her, and show her how awesome she could feel if she did some of these things that I'd done to turn my life around. I could tell she was living in a little bit of a cage that she didn't want to be in anymore, and I wanted to help set her free.

There was just one problem: the day before the dinner party, she informed me that she was deathly afraid of dogs. "My twin sister was backed into a corner by a huge, ferocious dog when we were both five, and I was completely helpless to save her, and even though nothing happened, she was fine, and I was fine, it stuck with me for the rest of my life," she said. "And it's bad. Like, sometimes I can't even move, like my whole body goes into paralysis when I'm close to a large dog."

"Wow. That's awful," I said.

"Is Peety a large dog?"

"He's fifty pounds, which technically is a medium-size dog. But he looks large to most people."

"Oh, God. OK. I just—"

"Look, text me when you get here. I'll bring him downstairs so you can meet each other outside. He's the sweetest dog ever, and I promise you guys will get along. I'm sure of it," I said.

I brought Peety downstairs when she arrived, and we met on the patch of lawn out in front of our building. I figured that was a lot safer than meeting in the apartment. If Peety sensed her fear there was no telling how he might interpret that, especially in his own castle.

Melissa looked like a scared child as we walked out. She stood nearly frozen, smiling a nervous smile.

"Hiiiii," she said.

"Hi," I said, pulling Peety back. He kept tugging on the leash trying to go greet her. "Go ahead and put your hand out like this, in sort of a fist, and put your head down, sort of looking at the ground, so he doesn't think you're trying to dominate him or anything, and then I'll let him come sniff your hand, OK?"

"Oh, God. OK," she said, and she put her hand out and looked at the ground and closed her eyes.

When Peety's wet nose touched her hand, she immediately pulled it back.

Peety wagged his tail and looked up at her, then over at me. I could tell he wanted to lick her.

"It's OK," I said. "Let him sniff it. He likes you, I can tell."

She put her hand back out, Peety licked it, and when she opened her eyes he started bouncing around all excited like he wanted to play.

"Oh, God, what's he doing?" she squealed, pulling her arms in tight across her chest.

I couldn't believe how high he was jumping. I'd seen him

do that a couple of other times when he got excited, too—literally jumping straight up in the air, higher than my head, again and again like he was bouncing on a giant pogo stick.

"He just wants to play! He likes you," I said. "All right, all right, Peety, Melissa's not ready to play yet, son. Let's give her a minute, OK?"

I walked him over to the bushes and let him go pee.

"All right, let's head in," I said.

"I'm so sorry," she said.

"No need to apologize. I appreciate you trying. Look, if any dog can turn you around, it'll be Peety. So no rush, OK?"

We rode up in the elevator together, and Peety kept looking up at Melissa the whole time.

"He *is* awfully cute," she said.

When the doors opened, Peety pulled me out and headed toward our door. I'm pretty sure he was excited to show the place off to our new friend. Melissa followed two steps behind us, and once we were inside, Peety circled around her a couple of times and tried to lead her into the living room, but then he decided to leave her alone. He lay down in front of the front door while we headed into the kitchen.

"Wow, your place is really nice," she said.

"Thank you."

"Oh, my gosh, I really like this tile."

"The backsplash? Yeah, isn't that cool? I did it myself."

"What? No way! So you cook, you do tile work—you're a regular renaissance man!"

"Ha, yeah. Maybe so," I said. "You ready to get started?"

"No. I'm afraid I'm going to ruin everything," she said. "I'm really not good in the kitchen."

"I promise you won't ruin a thing. This'll be fun."

On top of the paella, which we finished with smoked tempeh in an outdoor smoker that now stood proudly on my balcony, we put together a cocktail menu, and a big jug of sangria, and an array of Valencia-style "tapas" appetizers—from simple white olives, to a black-iron cornbread (which I sadly couldn't eat) made from stone-ground purple corn. Melissa took to it all like a pro. She was a really fast learner.

Melissa wasn't best friends with Peety at that point, but her extreme fright seemed to dissipate as the night went on. Peety didn't bug her. He wasn't all over her. But when she took a break and sat down at the kitchen table, he came over and lay down on her feet.

"That's a really good sign," I said to her.

"Yeah?"

"Yeah. He's basically giving you a hug."

"Oh," she said, looking down with a hesitant smile as she felt the warmth of his fur on her feet. "That's sweet."

The meet-up guest list that night was eclectic, including a physicist with a PhD; a gluten- and soy-free vegan in her thirties (who Melissa quietly insisted had her eyes on me, while I knew that my eyes were firmly fixed on Melissa); another guy named Syd who had helped Melissa start the meet-up group before we'd met; the two tech guys from India who showed up at every dinner; plus Melissa's twin sister and her boyfriend, who were vegetarian but not vegan and whom Melissa was hoping to persuade to go all the way.

The thing that struck me about Melissa is that she was an engaging host to everyone who walked through the door, and yet I didn't lose her to the party the way I used to lose Sarah. She stayed right with me, connected to me, as a partner and accomplice in making this whole dinner a great experience for everyone. We seemed to dance around each other in the kitchen, moving easily without bumping into each other—except when we did on purpose, with those sorts of little get-to-know-you touches that light up the senses. A hand on the small of the back as you scoot by each other, the touching of forearms as you reach for the bowl, that moment when I brushed the hair from her face for her while her hands were in the sink, and it took everything in me not to kiss her for the first time right there in front of our guests. I know she felt that longing, too. And a part of me could hardly wait for the dinner guests to leave.

Melissa's sister and brother-in-law were the last ones to go. I looked at the clock and it was 9:30 p.m. The two of us had spent nearly six hours together putting that whole party in motion from start to finish, and somehow every minute of the preparations and presentation had turned into something fun and engaging. I remember thinking, *Not for one second that entire afternoon or evening did things get tense or uncomfortable or awkward in any way.*

She was even coming around to getting more comfortable with Peety.

Sometimes you don't recognize what normal feels like until you feel it. And in those moments, you realize how maybe what you thought was normal in the past was really something less than what you wanted to feel.

Melissa was genuinely as nice a person as I'd ever spent time with, and I knew by the end of that party that I wanted to spend as much time with her as I could from that moment on.

When we closed the door, we both fell back against the walls of the hallway and let out a huge sigh of relief—then we laughed at our mutually timed sighs.

"That was *exhausting*!" she said.

"Yeah," I answered. "But good exhausting."

"Mmm-hmmmm," she agreed.

I couldn't wait another second. I stood up and put my right hand on the wall just above her shoulder. I leaned in, and I kissed her. Ever so gently.

It was perfect.

I looked in her eyes, and she looked in mine, and she lifted her hand to my neck to pull me in for a second kiss. Then we wrapped our arms around each other in a great big bear hug, when all of a sudden I felt her mouth open next to my ear—in a great big yawn!

"Ohhhhh," she said with a cute little laugh. "I'm so sorry. It's not you, I promise!"

"Maybe we should go sit down," I said.

She nodded.

I took her hand in mine, and as we turned to walk past the kitchen we both stopped and looked at the tremendous mess of dishes and pots and pans, spread across my countertops like the remnants of broken-down trucks and shell casings on a battlefield. Peety walked over and sat beside us as we leaned together in the doorway, and I saw Melissa reach down and gently pet him on the top of his head. I'm not even sure she was aware she did it, but it sure made me happy.

I suddenly found myself yawning, too, and I laughed. "Oh, man," I said. "Should we keep going and get that cleaned up now, before we sit down and don't want to get up again?"

Melissa thought about it for a moment as she leaned her head on my shoulder.

"Nah," she said. "Let's just wait and clean up in the morning."

# chapter 19

# On the Road

Melissa and I were pretty much inseparable after that first night. Within a week she was comfortable letting Peety snuggle right up next to her on the couch while we watched a movie. She stroked the back of his neck the whole time we sat there, and I was pretty sure he was already melting her heart.

Relationship-wise, after jumping in that first night, we took things kind of slow at first, at least by modern-day standards. We saw each other steadily for about a month before she introduced me to her children, one at a time.

She started with Joey, her six-year-old. "My calm, easy kid," she told me. Joey was deathly afraid of dogs, just like his mom, but we brought him over to meet Peety and walked him through the introduction, and in no time at all he was down on his knees on the floor and petting Peety's neck. It was awesome. He was a great kid who took after his mom, all full of energy and light and fun. And I think seeing his mom be OK around a dog for the first time really helped him get over his fear.

Melissa waited a few days to introduce me to her other son, Michael, though. She was worried. Michael was a preteen with autism. She told me that former boyfriends had sometimes found him difficult to be around. He might get upset about certain things, or shut down, or just be sort of antisocial at times, she said. Honestly, given who I was in my own past, I wasn't worried. I really liked Melissa and thought I'd be able to take it in stride. Plus, I had Peety the icebreaker—my conduit to the world.

Sure enough, Michael took to Peety right away. He liked dogs anyway, and had always wanted a dog of his own, so he and Peety got along like two brothers from day one. He would get right down on the floor and wrestle with Peety and let Peety lick his face, and that amazing relationship between the two of them served as the bridge that brought us all together.

Melissa wasn't ready to let Peety lick her face, even after a month or two, but Peety did his best to force her to like him. At times, when she and Michael were sitting on the couch, he would climb on top of them and lie across both of their laps with his full weight, preventing their escape and putting them on "lockdown" until they satisfied his demands for attention and petting.

Pretty much every day the five of us spent together, we grew closer, until finally it just felt annoying and wrong every time she and the boys left my condo.

"Maybe we should just move in together?" I said to her one day.

"Maybe we should," she said.

And just like that, Melissa and the boys moved into our condo. Peety and I suddenly had a family.

Being around me every day, sharing smoothies in the mornings and plant-based dinners every night, and coming along on my twice-a-day walks with Peety, Melissa began losing weight without even trying. The first time she realized she'd dropped five pounds, she was so excited about it that she decided to go all-in. She gave up vegan junk food and only ate my cooking. She stopped snacking on anything that came in a package. She basically tried to follow the same diet plan that had worked for me, and even started taking Peety out for walks by herself when I was gone for work.

I kept giving her cooking lessons, and she picked up the skills she needed to start cooking tasty meals for herself and her kids. And once she really grasped the concept of using spices to make even bland foods taste amazing, her kids fell in love with our way of eating, too. We all enjoyed whole-food, plant-based meals together as a family at our dining room table, every chance we got.

Within a few months, we were functioning like any other family. Work, school, homework, dinners, weekend play dates, day trips, and beach trips. Peety was in his glory. He had so much love to give, and now he had four times the people giving it back to him.

Following my plan, Melissa dropped from 210 pounds down to 135 in less than a year. She looked amazing. She went out shopping and came home feeling sexy. She wound up running outside with her boys and Peety, playing ball with them all and having the time of her life. The two of us grew closer than ever in the process, too.

But then something changed.

Melissa's new body and healthy lifestyle set her free— and she wanted to explore that freedom. She felt like she was seeing the world with new eyes, and she wanted to see the world from a new place. She started looking for new job opportunities, and the companies she wanted to work for weren't based anywhere in the Bay Area. She wanted to move. She wanted to start a whole new life, she said.

I felt uneasy about it from the start. I'd poured my heart and soul into fixing up my condo. I'd built a life with Peety, right where we were. I told her not to rush into anything. "Give it some time. Maybe we'll both feel that way at some point, by why rush things?" I said. We were happy. We had a great place to live. I thought my words were getting through to her.

Then one day she came home and told me she'd been offered a job—in Seattle.

"Well, if that's your choice, that's your choice," I said. "I just don't think I'm ready to move."

All of a sudden, it felt like everything we had built together was just a dream. I felt as if I'd been living in some sort of bubble, like a snow globe, and now I was on the outside of that bubble, looking in at a life that I once led. I couldn't grab hold of anything. I couldn't get back inside.

A few weeks later, I stood outside that glass and watched as Melissa and the boys packed their belongings into boxes. Then I helped them load it all onto a moving truck.

We didn't break up. We didn't really do anything. She told

me she hoped I would change my mind. She promised to call me to check in during their long drive north. I kissed her. I hugged her. I waved good-bye with tears in my eyes, and thought, *What the hell just happened?*

Sometimes, no matter how close we feel to someone, no matter how much they mean to us, we cannot know what they're really thinking, or feeling, or what they're going through on the inside. No matter how close we feel, we're all on our own journeys. We're all operating on our own clocks, in our own minds, from our own perspectives. And sometimes that makes it impossibly difficult to understand where we stand in this mixed-up world.

That night, I found myself eating dinner on the floor, just me and Peety, alone again, in our gorgeously decorated, completely empty apartment.

Melissa called the next night to let me know that she and the boys were OK. They were just getting ready to leave a roadside motel near the Oregon border. I thanked her for calling. I told her, "I love you," and she said, "I love you, too."

I cried myself to sleep in my room, holding Peety in my arms and realizing I'd made a huge mistake.

I called Melissa in the morning and told her I wanted to be together. I'd been a fool.

"Staying here doesn't make any sense. Where I live doesn't mean anything to me without *us*," I said.

She immediately broke down into tears. "Oh, my God, Eric, I'm so glad. I'm so glad. I don't want to do this without you," she said. "The boys are upset. They miss Peety. I miss Peety. I miss *you*."

When I got off the phone, I put the wheels in motion to sell the condo. I had already been looking to leave my job and move to a different employer. A new company I'd been exploring said they would try to accommodate me with a position anywhere I wanted to live. So I called them. They confirmed that I could work from Seattle. I took the job and said good-bye to my old company.

I ran the numbers and realized that by combining our resources, Melissa and I could afford to rent an unbelievable apartment in downtown Seattle, right in the center of everything, in a luxury building, with a panoramic view of the Seattle shipyards, and with a gym and a pool and a concierge. The cost of living in Seattle was so much less than it was in the San Francisco Bay Area. There's no income tax in Washington State, which meant I'd be giving myself a nearly 20 percent pay raise just by moving. I'd been a fool to not be open to Melissa's idea from the start.

My San Jose condo was a showplace, and I received an offer on it within a week. I did well on the sale. My new employer hired professional movers to move my stuff, and I decided to do something I'd never done in my life: rather than drive directly to Seattle and start work right away, I decided to take Peety on a road trip. I scheduled a weeklong vacation and plotted a loose course up the coast of California. Peety and I would hit the road for a weeklong adventure, stopping at every beautiful vista and cheesy tourist trap we could find between San Jose and Seattle.

It was impulsive. It was a little bit crazy. And it was going to be awesome.

The way I saw it, the two of us still had a lot of years to

make up for. We deserved to see the world, to take in the sights, and to do it at our own pace. I had vowed long ago that Peety would go places most dogs can't, and it was time to make good on that promise.

I searched Google Maps and came up with a basic route. We would drive all the way up the coast, from Northern California to Washington. I searched some travel sites, too, for potential destinations. I searched the web for all of the vegan-friendly restaurants and cafés I could find along the way. I made a list of them and plotted them along the map. It was only a loose plan, but when we were hungry, on almost any stretch of road, I knew I would be able to find us a good meal.

So off we went across the Golden Gate Bridge, stopping for our first vegan lunch at a little café in Sausalito.

From the moment we hit the road, it felt like Peety and I were making a leisurely transition between the old life we had and the new one ahead. All we felt was peace and freedom. It was mid-October. The skies were blue and the weather was clear; it wasn't scorching hot. And in some ways, making that transition felt like a bit of a re-birth.

A road trip leaves all sorts of time for reflection, and one of the things I thought about as we passed through Marin County was how I never would have made a trip like this by myself. If it was just me, I would have hopped on I-5 and sped up to Seattle in under two days flat. I had never gone to a movie by myself. I didn't like eating in restaurants by myself. Having a companion along for this ride allowed me to make it about *him*. I wanted to show Peety the sites along these roads. I was his personal chauffeur who just happened to get to enjoy the ride, too.

We weren't on the road for very long before I decided to make my first detour. Rather than head straight for the coast, I decided we ought to go see the wine country: Napa Valley. That whole region isn't that far north of San Francisco, and yet I'd never played tourist. I'd never been. It felt like a rite of passage, like walking the Golden Gate and going to Alcatraz. I had no idea when I'd be back this way after making the move to Seattle, so I threw caution to the wind and said, "Son, let's go get some wine."

We meandered east and pulled into Napa just in time to buy a ticket on the last Napa Valley Wine Train tour of the day. I never knew a Wine Train existed. We just followed some signs off the highway to see what it was, and wound up walking into this old-fashioned train-station building. Turns out they offered round-trip runs on this hundred-year-old train with dining cars and dessert cars, and that train took you out to a couple of different vineyards for tours of their wine-making facilities.

"Can the kitchen on the train accommodate a vegan?" I asked.

"The choices will be limited, but yes. Vegan, vegetarian, gluten-free—just tell your server once you get on board."

It was kind of expensive, but I said, "Why not? Sign us up!"

"I assume this is a service dog?" the man behind the ticket booth asked.

"He sure is," I said.

"OK."

Before we knew it, Peety and I were in line with people from all over the country and all around the world, some of whom had purchased tickets to this train ride months in advance. The fact that I just needed a single seat turned out to be a blessing. If I'd have brought another person along with me, I might not have been able to buy us tickets last-minute.

So Peety and I boarded the train—his first-ever train— and he lay right down under the table as the engine rumbled and the wheels started to turn. We rode through some gorgeous countryside, dotted with some of the world's most famous wineries. The vegan options on the menu were extremely few and far between. I didn't really eat enough food to make me full, which felt like a disappointment given the price they charged, but I didn't get upset about it. How could I be upset when I was sampling Napa wines on a nearly empty stomach?

Before long, Peety and I disembarked for our first tour, stepping into a world of wealth and taste the likes of which I was sure hardly a dog on earth had ever stepped a paw into. We marveled at the wines aging in row after row of oak barrels, and we enjoyed the pungent scent of fermenting grapes as the tour guide shared history we would never remember. I avoided buying wine or a "wine subscription" at the end of the tour, but I enjoyed some more samples regardless.

We then took a luxury coach bus to another vineyard and experienced the whole thing over again, only this time in a much more modern setting, filled with stainless-steel casks and a high-end gift shop, run by a flamboyant owner of French descent. I sampled some more wine, and this time I bought a bottle to bring to Melissa. We boarded the coach back to the train for the ride back to the station, and this time there was an empty seat next to me. So Peety hopped up on a fancy dining room chair and perched like a gentleman as he looked out the window the whole ride back.

With all of those wine samples in me and darkness approaching, we decided to call it a day. We didn't get far in miles, but we'd already experienced a day neither of us would ever forget. I thought it was a pretty good start.

The next day we headed north again up highway 101, and before long we were in redwood country. I decided to splurge for another train ride out into the forest, this time behind a big black locomotive engine that spewed steam into the air. It carried all of us passengers deep into the woods, and once we were there, we were allowed to get out and walk around those amazing trees. Peety loved it. It smelled so good, and the air was so clean. It felt magical, as if we would turn around and see gnomes hop out from the shadows and the thick greenery. Before we re-boarded for the trip back, I squatted down and tipped Peety's head toward the sky, right beside mine. "Look at that, boy. Look at how tall they are," I said.

Back on the road, we took the Redwood Highway, which sent us on a crazy winding hilly path through the forest, all the way out toward the ocean and US Route 1. Almost instantly the landscape changed from hills and forests to farmland to sprawling landscapes of pampas grass, with feathery plumes all waving in the breeze and catching the shimmer of the October sun.

When we grew tired, we found a motel and slept. When we got hungry, we looked for the nearest vegan-friendly restaurant and ate. I kept a bag of vegan food in the car, but most of the time we shared meals out, with my plate on the table and his on the ground. When we found ourselves driving up to a beautiful bluff, we stopped and got out and took in the scenery. When we spotted a sign for the famous "Drive-Thru Tree!" we spent five bucks to drive through it.

We turned into the parking lot of a theme park in the woods called Trees of Mystery, and decided not to take the gondola ride through the trees. But we did take the time to marvel at their giant statues of Paul Bunyon and Babe the Blue Ox while Peety answered the call of nature.

We stopped in little downtown areas in tiny towns with names I would never remember, and we wandered in and out of shops full of oddball items. We watched waves crashing into the rocks and marveled at every sunset.

The length of the California coast north of San Francisco is staggering. If you believe what they show in movies and what they teach for geography in most schools, you'd think the top of California is just north of the Napa Valley. But it goes on and on beyond that.

We stopped in Santa Rosa, California, just to tip our hat to the birthplace of Amy's Organics, which grew from a tiny idea into one of the biggest and certainly most recognizable all-natural food companies in the world. We spent the night at a hotel in nearby Ukiah. And then we finally crossed into Oregon and headed for Eugene—the birthplace of the American jogging movement.

Eugene is the city where Nike got its start. It's still headquartered there. And Eugene is really the birthplace of running as a popular pastime in the United States. It felt so cool to spend a day in that city. And even though Peety wasn't big on running, I took him for a short jog on one of the trails in town, just to say we did it.

That afternoon, we stopped by the Cornbread Café, which is a roadside diner except for one unique fact: it's completely vegan. They serve all sorts of diner and greasy-spoon staples, but with no meat or dairy whatsoever. The comfort food there is so ridiculously tasty, Guy Fieri once featured it on his TV show, *Diners, Drive-Ins and Dives*—a show that usually shows off rib shacks and places that serve three-pound hamburgers.

Before we knew it, we were approaching the Washington State border.

Peety seemed a little down during the final stretch of that trip. I'm not sure if it settled in that we weren't going to be going back to our old home, or if maybe we'd just been away from Melissa and the kids for so long that he missed their company. Maybe he was sad that the trip was almost over. Or perhaps dogs go into periods of deep reflection like we humans do. I'm not sure. I know I spent a lot of our quiet time on those long stretches of road thinking about all the things Peety and I had done and seen together over the last four years. It was staggering how much each of our lives had changed.

Or maybe he was just tired from all of that traveling. I know I was.

I was ready to go home. To our new home. To start a whole new life in a new city. There would be so much to explore and so much to discover, I wondered in some way if it would feel like this road trip was ongoing—as if our lives had now transformed into a never-ending adventure.

I knew one thing for sure: I wanted to do everything I could to make sure Peety's new home was comfortable and happy for him, and the best place he'd lived in his whole life.

# chapter 20

# Homeward Bound

Life on the fourteenth floor was pretty great for Peety and me. Peety had his patch of grass in the sky and was glad to be back with his family. I was glad to be back with them, too. Harbor Steps (in prime zip code 98101) was one of the nicest settings I'd ever called home, smack in the middle of absolutely everything a person could ever want. We were two blocks away from Pike Place Market with its rows and rows of fresh produce available daily; a couple of blocks up from a magnificent waterfront; diagonally across from the art museum; literally steps away from great restaurants and three coffee shops on our block alone.

Our building had a pool, a pool table, a library, a Jacuzzi, a gym, an indoor basketball court, and an outdoor courtyard with a fountain where Peety and I could relax and take a quiet lunch now and then. Melissa's job was located in a high-rise right across the street, which meant we could grab lunch together on days when I worked from home.

There was a Whole Foods nearby, and just a few miles

out of town Peety and I discovered an oasis called Green Lake Park—a beautiful lake surrounded by a 2.2-mile walking path adjacent to a big off-leash, fenced-in dog run. Just a couple of blocks from there we discovered a place called the Wayward Café, too, a comfort-food vegan place sort of like the Cornbread Café in Eugene, except three times as big and with an even broader menu.

It quickly became clear to me that Seattle was one of the most dog-friendly cities in the country, and the most vegan-friendly town I had seen since Berkeley. I started to wonder if perhaps dogs and vegans went hand-in-hand.

Funny enough, I found that most runners I met were dog lovers as well.

For some reason, everywhere I looked, dogs and healthy lifestyles and happy people seemed to go paw in hand.

Seattle was truly a fresh start for me. For all of us. Everything seemed new. Everything seemed refreshing. It felt good to be by the water. It was fun for the kids to be in the middle of a tourist district, too. We were down the street from the Hard Rock Cafe, and blocks away from the Seattle Great Wheel—the gargantuan Ferris wheel that rivals the Eye in London. And of course Seattle was also home to the famous Space Needle. We explored all of those places, not only with the boys but also with Peety. So Peety literally rode up into the sky and looked out over the whole city from all of these amazing man-made vantage points.

I also found a little beach along my running path where Peety could wade safely into the Puget Sound. And he occasionally had a chance to splash in the lake and send a few ducks flying up into the air at the park. He truly had every amenity and excursion a dog could ever want available at his paw tips. Even the staff at the concierge desk fell in love with Peety. They always greeted him with a great big smile and had treats for him at the ready.

And of course we continued our tradition of morning and afternoon walks, no matter what other activities we got up to. Eating right and taking those two, thirty-minute walks each day were the routine that made all of this possible. I would never forget that. And neither would Peety.

Work got a bit busier for me as I settled into my new job, though. I found I had to fly out of town a little more often than with my previous company. My sales territory was spread out over a wider area than before, which meant that I had more plane flights and overnight trips.

It bothered me that I couldn't bring Peety with me on my trips. I sometimes kicked myself for not trying to train him to come with me to airports and have the patience to fly with me on planes. He'd done so well on our train trips in California, I wondered if maybe I'd unnecessarily feared how he might do on flights. But it seemed a little late to try to find out now. Plus, while I sometimes worried about having another blackout, I hadn't suffered another in all that time—despite the fact that I was running more often than ever and entering more marathons than ever before. I figured it was safe enough to travel without him.

I also felt more comfortable leaving Peety with Melissa and the boys. They loved him, and he always seemed like he was in heaven with his family all around him. The bonus for me was I always enjoyed a beautiful homecoming after every trip. As soon as he heard my keys, Peety would come flying across the room to greet me at the front door of our apartment with a series of high-bouncing, joyful doggie leaps in the air.

It was funny, though. As spring approached, I came home from one trip and noticed that Peety didn't do his usual leaps. He ran to me. He spun in circles. He was as excited as ever. But he didn't leap.

That night in bed, I asked Melissa, "Does Peety seem any different to you?"

"What do you mean?"

I told her about my greeting, and she said, "Well, come to think of it, he's been moving a little bit slower on his walks."

"Has he?" I said. I hadn't noticed that.

"Yeah. Just a little. I don't know. Maybe I'm wrong."

"Huh," I said. I really didn't think anything of it. He was eating fine and didn't show any other signs of being sick or injured. He was current on all of his shots. Everything seemed fine at his last checkup, which was just before I left San Jose—so only four or five months earlier. He had a mobile grooming service here that came around and kept him looking sharp, too, and they hadn't mentioned anything out of the ordinary.

"Maybe he's just starting to show his age a little," I said.

"How old is he now, anyway?" Melissa asked.

"I'm not telling," I said.

"Oh, like you wouldn't tell me you were *fifty-four* when we first started dating?" she said.

I laughed.

"Yeah. Real funny."

"You thought I was forty-three!" I said, still laughing.

"Nah, I was just stroking your ego. I figured you were sixty-something," she joked.

"Oh, really?" I said.

"Yeah!" she said.

"Oh, really?!"—I grabbed her and started tickling her, and Peety moaned at us from the foot of the bed.

"Stop it!" Melissa said. "I have to work in the morning. Go to sleep. Peety's tired, too."

"All right, all right," I replied.

I turned out the light, and in the darkness, I told her, "He's twelve. He could even be close to thirteen. He was seven-something when I got him, so...yeah. At least twelve."

"Hmm," she said. "Well, good night."

"Good night," I whispered. "Good night, Peety."

It was just a couple of weeks later, in the second week of March, when I took Peety out for a late walk around the neighborhood. That's when I noticed he was walking a bit slower when we left the building. That's also when he saved my life in spectacular fashion—by leaping six feet in the air to defend me from that aggressive panhandler who emerged from the shadows on the corner of Pike and Second.

Two days later, I left on yet another business trip. This time I had to go to Dallas for a trade show. It was early evening on the first night when I got the call from Melissa.

"Eric," she said. I could hear the quaver in her voice the moment she started speaking. "There's something wrong with Peety."

"What do you mean?"

"He's sick. He's not eating. He barely wants to get up, even for Michael," she said.

"Oh, no. Something he ate? Did he get into something?"

"I don't know. He's not acting like himself at all."

"You remember the sprout incident, right?" I asked her.

As part of my quest to eat ever-fresher, more nutrient-dense food, I started growing my own sprouts in San Jose. One day, Peety got into my package of organic broccoli seeds. He ripped into them and ate at least a cup of them. He wound up having diarrhea near the creek at Penitencia Creek Park the next morning, and several weeks later, a patch of fresh organic broccoli started growing in the spot. We laughed at the fact that Peety had not only planted broccoli, but also fertilized it!

"No, I don't think it's anything like that," Melissa said. "There's nothing torn apart anywhere, nothing open, nothing."

The fact that she didn't laugh at the broccoli-seed memory made me wonder what kind of shape Peety was in.

"Maybe you'd better take him to the vet," I said.

"It's late. They're closed," she said.

"Well, take him first thing in the morning. Or take him to an emergency vet. Put it on my credit card," I said.

"OK," she replied. "I'll let you know."

"OK. Give him a kiss for me."

I had meetings the next day. Melissa texted and said the vet wanted to keep Peety overnight for observation. I thought about flying back early, but I had an important dinner party to attend that night at the Gaylord Texan, a fancy, Texas-size hotel and convention complex. It was my first year at this new job. I felt like leaving to take care of my sick dog wouldn't go over too well, and Melissa agreed. "There's nothing you can do," she said. "I'll go back in the morning."

We were just wrapping things up at the dinner when I got a text alert on my phone, warning me of a large charge on my credit card. It was for veterinary services in the amount of $1,800. I called Melissa on the way back to my hotel room and she said they ran a whole battery of tests, an MRI, and more, and that we should have results the next day.

I was at a business breakfast the next morning when my phone rang. It was Melissa. I excused myself and stepped out into a quiet hallway.

"Hey, what's up?" I said. "How's Peety."

Melissa was crying.

"You've got to fly home, Eric. He's not well. He's not well at all," she said.

"What do you mean? What is it?"

"They said...they said they found a massive growth on his spleen."

I felt faint. I could barely stand up. I had to lean myself against the wall.

"What?" I said.

"He could barely walk. We had to get help lifting him into the car. Poor Michael had to lift him out and carry him to the apartment, Eric. He's not moving. He still hasn't touched any food or water," she said.

"Wait—they sent him home?"

"Yes, Eric," she said. "They said no matter what it is, it's massive. And..."

"And what?"

"They don't think he's gonna make it."

"What?"

I started to cry. Someone opened a door to the restaurant, and the sound of diners talking and eating and scraping forks on plates seemed deafening to me.

"Just…take care of him, OK? Take care of him. I'm sure they're wrong. I'm positive. I'm going to see if I can catch a flight and get out of here today."

"Try, sweetie. Please. I can't do this alone. I can't."

"Just tell him I'll be home as soon as I can. Tell him. He understands, OK? Tell him."

I couldn't get a flight out until the afternoon. It was a connecting flight. There was a delay at the second airport and the wait nearly tore me apart. I wanted to scream. It was evening by the time I arrived in Seattle. I told the cab to hurry. "*Please.*"

I opened the front door of our apartment expecting the sound of Peety's paws to come scurrying across the floor.

They didn't.

"Hello?" I called.

"Over here," Michael said.

I followed the sound of his voice toward the balcony, where I found Michael on the floor with one arm wrapped around Peety, both of them lying on top of a neatly laid cushion of piled-up blankets. The balcony door was open, filling the room with fresh night air. Melissa came out of the bedroom.

"Joey's asleep. He was up all last night," she whispered.

I caught a glimpse of Joey in the bed behind her.

Peety didn't stand up. He didn't even raise his head. He looked at me with his big beautiful eyes, and I completely lost it. I fell to my knees and started bawling my eyes out.

"Peety, what's up, son?" I said, kissing his forehead. "What's the matter, boy?"

Michael sat up as I lay next to my boy and pulled my whole body around him.

"Has he eaten at all?" I asked.

"No," Melissa said.

"Anything?"

"No water, either. We wet a washcloth and squeezed a little in his mouth. We tried giving him spoonfuls of water, and he lapped them up at first, but then he stopped. It's been hours. We've tried everything."

"Did the vet call back with any news?"

"No. I called over again but apparently the test results didn't go out, or something. The fax machine was broken? I don't know. That place was completely disorganized."

"What?"

"It…they just didn't know what they were doing. Did you see how much they charged?"

"Yeah. I don't care about the money. I just…"

I didn't want to argue. I didn't want to get mad. I just wanted my boy to feel better.

"They didn't give any suggestions about what to do?" I said.

"They gave me a number for an animal hospice service, Eric. That's the only thing they gave me."

I could barely breathe. I tried to take some deep breaths and think. There had to be something more we could do.

That's when I noticed how slow and shallow Peety's breaths were.

"My God," I said. "I'm right here, boy. I'm right here. How could this happen so out of the blue?"

"I don't know," Michael said.

Joey sat up in the bed. "Is Peety gonna be all right?" he called.

"I don't know, kiddo. I just don't know."

"We tried taking him onto the balcony," Michael said, "'cause he hasn't gone to the bathroom in forever, but he wouldn't go. He wouldn't stand up. I wanted him to have some fresh air, so I stayed here with him."

"You did good, Michael. You did great."

The air was a little chilly, so I decided to move Peety into the bedroom. I grabbed the edge of the blankets and slid him across the floor, right next to our bed. I lay down, exhausted from the flights and the panic of wanting to get home. I dangled one arm over the side so I could keep petting him. Melissa was lying down beside me, and Joey and Michael were both lying on the floor with their arms on Peety.

"I just can't believe this," I said. "How could this happen. Why? Why now? Why?"

Peety let out a moan, and I started to cry again.

"Maybe we should turn the light out," Melissa said.

"Yeah. That's a good idea. Let's everyone get some rest," I said.

Melissa got up and turned off the light, and Peety let out a whimpering cry unlike anything I'd ever heard from him before.

"What's the matter, boy? What is it?" I said.

Melissa turned the light back on and he stopped. We all petted him until he calmed down again. But when she tried to turn the light off, he started whimpering again.

"No, turn it back on," I said.

I climbed down on the floor and put my arm around him. "Try leaving the bathroom light on," I said. She did, and when she turned the overhead light off, the light from the bathroom seemed to give Peety comfort. He wanted to be able to see and didn't want to be alone.

"I wish there were something I could do," I said.

"Me, too," said Michael.

"Me, three," said Joey.

Melissa asked the boys to come up in bed with her and get some rest. I stayed right next to Peety, and I quietly sang him his favorite John Lennon song.

"Now it's time to say good night, good night, sleep tight. Now the sun turns out his light, good night, sleep tight…"

I stayed on the floor with Peety all night. His breathing grew heavy. Every once in a while he'd let out a big sigh. I closed my eyes for long stretches and then jerked myself awake in a panic, making sure he was still with us. Each time I did that, Peety looked at me. And every time he looked at me, I teared up.

Peety made it through the night. But his breathing grew more labored. Melissa placed a call to the hospice. If there was any way to make him more comfortable, we wanted to know how to do that. They told us that someone would be there within a couple of hours.

We kept the boys home from school. Melissa called in

sick to work. I didn't even bother calling in. I didn't want to move from Peety's side for even one second.

"Why don't you at least get some water or something. Stretch your legs. You've been in one place all night," Melissa said to me.

"Stay right with him?" I said.

"Of course," she said, and she and the boys all got down on the floor and gently laid their hands on Peety's back.

I went to the bathroom and then walked out to get myself a cup of water. When I came back in the room, I lay down on the floor, put my hand on Peety's neck, and scratched him behind the ears.

Peety looked me right in the eyes.

"It's OK, son," I said. "It's OK. I'm right here."

Seconds later, he let out a big, long breath. His body shuddered as his spirit left him. I watched the light in his eyes go out.

It was as peaceful as could be.

I had never watched an animal die before, and for a moment I was relieved that it didn't seem painful. I was grateful to know that I was right there with him, and thankful that he was surrounded by people he loved, and who loved him.

For a moment.

And then it hit me.

My dog. My boy. My son. My heart.

My Peety.

Was gone.

# chapter 21

# A New Hope

An hour or so later, Dr. Jason Goodwin from the pet hospice knocked on our door.

He wheeled a cart into our apartment.

He was kind and compassionate and gentle with his words.

He asked us whether we wanted to have Peety's ashes returned to us, or whether we were planning a burial. I said no to both.

He brought some molding clay into the bedroom and took impressions of Peety's paw prints. That clay would serve as the basis of a memorial plaque that I would create to remember Peety and later be very grateful to have. But at the time, any of those sorts of funeral rituals seemed unimportant to me. Nothing could possibly reflect or honor or come close to memorializing Peety, what he had done, what he meant, or who he was. Nothing.

After wrapping Peety's body and placing it on the cart, Dr. Goodwin wheeled it across our floor. I knew that

body was no longer Peety. Peety was gone. I had watched
him go.

Dr. Goodwin took the time to close the door gently behind him as he left. He turned the handle before it closed so
it barely made a click.

I appreciated that.

We all sat there in the awful quiet of that apartment, re-
treating to a chair or a sofa or a bed; taking bites of whatever
fruit or nut seemed tolerable enough to swallow; squinting
out at the reflected sun as it glistened and rippled on Puget
Sound; staring at an empty patch of grass that now seemed
without purpose so high in the sky.

The boys would both shed tears that night as we tucked
them into bed.

Melissa would cry as she fell asleep.

But not me. I felt empty and seemed to be all cried out.

As my first sleepless night wore on, I felt a gnawing, acidic
clench in my stomach that I hadn't felt in nearly five years.

In the morning, the boys would go to school. Melissa
would go to work. And I would sit alone in the apartment—
and eat.

I ate leftover rice and beans until it was gone. I ate up all
of our fruit and some nuts. An hour later, I was hungry again.

I didn't want to talk to anyone about Peety, so before the
kids got home, I went out. I left a note saying I didn't know
what time I'd be back. I wandered all over downtown Seattle. I walked, and walked, with no direction. I stopped in
a little Mexican joint and ordered a veggie taco in a fresh-
made corn tortilla. It tasted incredible, so I ordered six more.
I did not care what those tortillas might do to my body.

I started walking again and still felt that gnawing in my stomach, so I stopped in a convenience store. I walked out with two containers of Coconut Bliss ice cream, one of the many accidentally vegan snacks to be found on America's junk food shelves. I ate them both.

I stopped into the Hard Rock Cafe. I appreciated the loudness of the music. I sat at the bar alone and drank bourbon. I downed more bourbon than I'd downed since I was a soldier in Germany. I drank in silence until the bartender told me he had to cut me off.

I stumbled around the corner, felt the rush of the elevator as I stumbled my way to the fourteenth floor, and opened the apartment door to nothing but darkness and the lack of a greeting. I fell into bed.

"God, Eric. You reek!" Melissa said.

I groaned at her and passed out.

When I woke, the clench in my stomach was still there. I wanted to make it stop. I didn't crave meat or anything far outside of the diet I'd been feeding myself for the last five years. I wouldn't dishonor Peety's memory in that way. I certainly would not stray from the ethical side of my diet. Ever. But the healthy side? I wondered why it mattered anymore.

I ate, and ate, and ate. At a Thai restaurant, alone in a corner, I devoured three whole dishes meant to serve four people each. The waiter laughed.

"Wow! You hungry!"

I didn't crack a smile.

"Yes," I said. "I am."

A couple of days later I went back to work. I purposefully

took on more travel. I ate airport food and drank at airport bars.

I went home and felt like Melissa was a stranger. I felt disconnected from her kids. I found myself getting frustrated at Michael more than in the past.

Three months went by, and the hurt didn't stop. Then, things suddenly turned. Our affordable nine-month lease ran out on us, and the building sent us a renewal bill. They jacked up our rent by more than a thousand dollars per month. It was too much. Melissa was making a decent salary, but not enough to cover the difference, and my sales had slipped since Peety died, which left us no choice but to move. We found a cheap rental in the suburbs. It was small. It was run-of-the-mill housing. We squeezed ourselves into it and learned to live without the amenities and conveniences money can buy.

Melissa now had to commute, which meant she had to buy her own car. The additional financial stress upset her. "Most people in this country have to buy a car in order to work at their jobs, Melissa. It's not some crazy, unusual thing," I told her. Still, she complained. Every day. About the drive. About the expense of gas. She was absolutely blown away by the cost of car insurance. Somehow, this was my fault.

It became glaringly obvious to me just how many years there were between us.

I was miserable to live with after Peety was gone. I recognized that. I didn't want to socialize. I merely wanted to do my work and spend quiet nights at home. I couldn't face the world without him. I thought Melissa, of all people, would understand that.

But she didn't seem to understand.

She kept bugging me to go out. She kept bugging me to let her invite some people over. She wanted to "hang out," she said.

"Hang out? What does that even mean?" I said meanly.

She stormed out to go spend a night on the town with some people from work.

I felt as if I didn't want to spend a night on the town with anybody ever again. *I'm too old for this crap.*

Six months passed, all a fog, all one blur, and in those months I packed on between twenty and thirty pounds, depending on which scale I stepped on.

I started to feel sick. I had chest pains that may or may not have been acid reflux. I took that as a sign. I decided I'd better get a checkup. I thought, *Maybe these chest pains mean it's time I try to get out of this funk.*

I made an appointment with a doctor I'd never met, at Virginia Mason Hospital in Seattle, and when I walked in, what I saw at the receptionist's desk stopped me cold. This woman had a photo of a dog pinned to the side of the cubicle next to her computer—a dog who looked just like Peety.

"Is that your dog?" I asked.

"*Was* my dog, yes. She's been gone a couple of years now," she said.

"I'm sorry," I said.

"Thank you. She was a great dog."

"Yeah. I bet. I had a dog who looked just like that."

"Really?" she said.

"A boy. Peety. I lost him a few months ago. I can't seem to get over it."

"I'm so sorry to hear that. I'm still not over mine. Not really, anyway. I'm not sure I'll ever get over her being gone," she said.

"But you're functioning, right? I'm, like, barely functioning. I mean—how did you do it? How did you get back to some sense of normalcy?"

"I got a new dog," she said. "That helped."

She showed me a picture. The new dog didn't look anything like Peety.

"Oh," I said. "I don't think I could do that."

"Give it some time," she said. "If your dog meant that much to you, then I have a feeling you'll find another. Actually, it works the other way: when there's a dog out there who's trying to find you, you'll know it."

"What do you mean?"

"When your dog is out there trying to find you, you'll know it. Your old dog will help you, and you'll just know it," she said.

I felt a chill run through my body. It was one of the weirdest conversations I'd ever had. Who was this woman? I couldn't stop thinking about it. I left my appointment that day and didn't even get her name, and yet the notion that a dog might be out there, "looking for me," kept rattling around in my mind. I couldn't let it go.

I told Melissa about it, and she thought we ought to go look at some local shelters just to see if maybe there was a dog that was "looking for me." But she also made it pretty clear that she wasn't too keen on getting another dog. She didn't want to have to take care of it. She knew I did most of the work, though, and she wanted to support me.

So we stopped into shelters all over the region. We saw some really cute dogs, but I didn't feel instantly connected to any of them. None of them seemed to be "my dog." None of them seemed to be looking for me.

As we did that, I came to realize how completely unique the process of adopting a dog at Humane Society Silicon Valley had been. None of these other shelters had a matchmaker like Casaundra. Most other shelters just let people pick out the dog they thought they wanted. It seemed so strange to me. Without Casaundra, I never would have picked Peety—and Peety was the dog I really needed, who needed me, who was perfect for me.

I kept popping into shelters every few days for the next couple of weeks in some vague hope that I'd suddenly be overcome with a feeling that one of those dogs was looking for me. Eventually I just started to feel foolish. *Why did I listen to that woman anyway?*

At home, I sat on the couch for long stretches and felt the absence of Peety's head on my lap. I missed his warmth on my feet under the breakfast table. I missed his presence in the backseat of my car.

I no longer took walks in the morning and evenings.

I didn't know how to walk without him.

Then one day, I set my alarm and got up early to run the Seattle Marathon Association's annual 10K race. I had pretty much stopped running, but I'd registered for this race months earlier, and I decided I ought to follow through on my commitment. I didn't pay a whole lot of money to enter, but still: I didn't like to waste money, and once I was committed to something, I liked to follow through on it. Plus, it was only 6.2 miles; I could do that in my sleep.

So I ran it. Completely out of practice and out of shape, while carrying an extra 15 percent of my body weight, I finished. I had barely slowed down and had just bent over with my hands on my hips—trying to catch my breath—when a feeling washed over me like I'd never felt before: I felt that there was a dog out there trying to find me. I felt it as clearly as I felt the throbbing in my knees and the soles of my feet.

I hopped in my car and drove straight to the closest shelter: Seattle Humane Society.

Seattle Humane wasn't a modern facility like HSSV. They had signs up announcing a new facility soon to be under construction, but the current facility was no more than a concrete, white-painted, low-slung building. The structure was surrounded by trees, with a tiny parking lot, and with rows of kennels from which I could hear dogs barking as I exited my car.

Walking through the lobby, I was struck by the pungent smell of disinfectant, and I was glad to get out the back door into the open courtyard between the main building and the kennels. I didn't talk to anyone. I didn't ask anyone for help. I just walked directly toward the kennels, which featured a painted sign that said, "Adoption Dorms." I opened the door and stepped inside a long hallway with dogs in pens on either side. I looked into the first kennel on the left, and then on the right. I stepped forward, and in the second kennel on the left, there he was: a jet-black Labrador retriever, thin, tall, young, fit, sturdy, and with the kindest eyes. All of the other dogs were barking up a storm and jumping around, but not this one. This one stood there, confident, and he looked right at me, like he knew me. He looked into my eyes as if he were saying, "Dude, what took you so long? Let's get out of here!"

He didn't have an information sheet on his kennel door like the other dogs down the row. I didn't know his name. There were no volunteers in there at the time, but I didn't want to leave and risk someone else coming in to claim him. I walked to the door to the courtyard, opened it only halfway, and hollered to the first volunteer I saw: "Hey, can I please get a hand in here?"

The young lady walked over and I told her, "I'm really interested in this dog."

"Willy? OK, wow. We just brought him in here like four minutes ago. I haven't even had a chance to print out his information yet. Hold on and I'll go get it for you."

*Willy?* That name did not fit this dog at all.

When she came back I asked her, "Why Willy? Is that the name he came in with?"

"No, he was a stray. They picked him up. He'd been living in the wild, no collar, no chip, so they held him for fourteen days. They put notices out. But no one claimed him. So they cleaned him up, had him neutered, brought him here this morning. He just looked like a Willy to one of the staff," she said. "You want to get to know him a little bit?"

"Yeah, if I could," I said.

She led Willy and me both through the courtyard to a small fenced-in, get-to-know-you pen, with a bench where I could sit, and a rope toy and a hard rubber ball, and she left us alone. Willy came over to me immediately and put his head right into my lap, just like Peety used to do. I scratched him behind his ears. He kept looking up at me, directly into my eyes. I swear he was urging me with his look and begging me to take him home.

I picked up the rope toy and he went right for it. I spun it around over his head and he spun right around and followed its every move, eventually lunging and grabbing it in his strong jaw, playfully pulling and not letting go as I lifted his front legs right off the ground.

"OK, drop it," I said, and he immediately let go.

"Sit," I said, and he sat.

"Down," and he went down.

This was not a wild dog.

I tossed the rubber ball, and he chased it down and brought it right back to me. I had to wrestle to get it out of his mouth, but then he sat down and barked at me, like, "Throw it again! Throw it again!"

This dog was awesome! I couldn't understand it. He was well trained. He was fit. He was *beautiful*. Had he gotten lost? Or had someone taken him out into the woods and let him go?

I took a picture with my phone and sent it to Melissa. "I found my dog," I said. "What do you think?"

Her response was, "Well, it's your dog."

I texted back, "Yeah, I know it's my dog. But what do you think?"

"It's OK with me. Do whatever you want," she said.

It was so disappointing. I had never felt more disconnected from her than in that moment. Here I was on the precipice of a major decision, feeling as if I'd completed a long hard journey and finally found my buried treasure, truly feeling as if I might be ready to get back into life, and it felt as if she didn't care.

A part of me wondered how much longer our relationship would last.

"So." The volunteer's voice startled me as I put my phone away. "How are you two doing?" she asked from the other side of the fence.

"We're doing great," I said. "What do you think, boy?"

Willy cocked his head to the side and stared at me before putting his head on my knee.

"You want to go home?"

"Woof!" he barked, and he stood up and circled around and around in front of the gate, just itching to get out and go. I couldn't help but think that the woman in the doctor's office had been absolutely right. This had Peety written all over it. He helped me find this dog. He helped this dog find *me*.


After filling out some paperwork I took Willy outside, and he hopped into the back of my car like we were on our way home from a hike or run. He sat down in the backseat and tried to climb over into the front only one time on the whole ride home. All it took was me putting my arm up and saying, "No. Sit, boy, sit," and he sat for the rest of the ride.

I thought about what to name him as I drove, but I still wasn't sure.

The boys were real excited to meet him when I got home. They threw their arms around him, and he seemed to handle all of that attention and touching just fine.

"I'm thinking I might call him Luther," I said.

"What?!" Michael yelled.

"No way!" Joey said.

"I think his name is Jake," Michael said.

"Jake?" I replied.

"Yes, Jake," he said. "Like the other dog I knew."

"Oh," I said. I looked to Melissa, wondering what other dog he might be talking about, but she just shrugged her shoulders.

"Well, let me think about it," I said.

"No!" Michael insisted. "His name is Jake. Jake is his name."

I actually really liked the sound of it. I would have liked to have known the story about why Michael insisted on that name for him, but I never got it out of him.

"Jake," I said. "All right. Jake it is."

There was something about Jake's frame that looked like a runner's build to me. I had visions of him living in the wild, chasing down his food and surviving for God knows how long after being lost or abandoned, and I wondered if he'd like to go for a run with me. So the next morning I woke up early, tied up the laces on my New Balance running shoes, and brought Jake out to one of my favorite short trails at Bridle Trails Park in Kirkland. It's about a four-mile loop. I thought it would be an easy enough start. If he didn't like the running, I figured we could take a nice walk together at the very least.

Jake kept trying to chase squirrels as we walked to the trailhead. He yanked on the leash so hard I felt like he was going to pull my arm out of its socket.

*Great*, I thought. *This isn't going to work at all.*

But as soon as I got on the trail and started running, Jake fell in line right next to me. He didn't pull on the leash, he didn't stray from the path, and he even ignored the squirrels. We passed other runners and he didn't bark at them. We passed another runner with a dog, and he started to stray to go sniff that dog out, but with a gentle pull on the leash he fell right in line at my side and we kept on running.

We rounded the whole loop without a hitch.

"Good boy, Jake!" I said, squatting down and petting him, and looking into those beautiful eyes.

"Woof!" he barked, pulling back toward the trail as if he wanted to run it again.

"No, no, that's enough for today. Let's start slow, OK? We'll build up to it."

I went home and researched running for dogs, and I found a whole new world to explore. It turns out Labs are extremely good runners who can cover miles and miles with ease. I worried that running long distances might be damaging to his paws or his joints, but I found all kinds of evidence from vets and other pet owners suggesting that dogs were able to run marathons, just like we humans were, if properly trained.

There were even special dog-and-human races out there we could participate in when we were ready.

As I continued to scan the web for information, Jake snuggled himself right up next to me on the couch. I could hardly believe how bonded the two of us seemed after just one day. I scratched the top of his head and thought about Peety, and felt crushingly sad. I hoped he didn't feel I was betraying him by moving on like this and bonding with a new dog.

But then Jake looked up at me with a familiar look in his eye. He gave me that look that only a dog can give—a look of unconditional love, as if I, in my slightly out-of-shape, still depressed and overweight state, was somehow the greatest guy in the whole world, just because I took him home and decided to share my life with him.

Seeing that look, I knew that Peety was there with us. He wasn't just OK with this. He wanted this for me. Because the last thing he ever wanted was to see me sad.

I was right about my relationship with Melissa. She was unhappy. She said she didn't want us to be together anymore. She asked me and Jake to move out.

Her kids didn't seem surprised. I guess they were somewhat expecting it. I don't know. I hoped the breakup wouldn't scar either of them in any way. And I remember thinking that maybe we'd moved too quickly. Maybe we should have slowed things down. Maybe we should have looked at the age difference between us and realized there was just no way we would remain compatible for the long haul.

I don't know. It's hard not to second-guess everything when things go wrong.

All I knew was that it was over. I was very glad I had Jake in my life before it ended, because moving out to yet another apartment entirely on my own would have been a lot harder without my new pal.

Jake and I started running every day. After taking him to

a veterinarian for a checkup and consultation, I put him on a high-protein plant-based diet, and before long, he was building muscle and running like a champion.

Having him in my life made my life feel complete again, and I decided I needed to honor that in every way possible. I decided that I was going to become a true animal welfare activist, and I was going to show my love for animals in every choice I made.

When we moved into our new apartment, I sold or donated every piece of leather furniture I had. I donated my leather shoes and my cowboy boots to Goodwill, and I replaced them with vegan-friendly shoes—made from non-animal-based materials, including some really nice-looking dress shoes made from recycled tires. People are always shocked when I tell them, because they look just like fine leather. I stopped wearing leather belts and threw out my leather wallet. I paid more attention to avoid any hair products or soaps from companies that test products on animals. I went full-contact vegan. I wanted every facet of my life to reflect my beliefs, and my beliefs were based in kindness.

I also trained Jake to act as my service dog, just like Peety had, and I made up my mind that I would really take him everywhere I went. I regretted not taking Peety on every business trip. I regretted every minute I didn't spend with that beautiful dog. I wasn't about to have those same regrets with Jake. So the next time I had a business trip scheduled, I took Jake flying with me, riding in the passenger cabin. He curled himself up at my feet and didn't bother a soul on that plane. In fact, he gave people all sorts of smiles. Grumpy children and their beleaguered moms, uptight businessmen and overworked flight attendants alike couldn't help but smile, seeing that great big beautiful dog get onto the plane with his service-dog collar tag.

Living my beliefs fully has made me a kinder person. Expressing my passions for the causes I believe in, dedicating myself to running and eating well, have made me happier than I've ever been in my life. And oddly enough, giving myself to these causes, donating my time and even my money to make the world a better, kinder, gentler place, has somehow resulted in me receiving more love and generosity in return than I ever thought possible. I've even become a better salesman. And I give so much of the credit for all of that to Peety, and now to Jake.

Just like Peety, Jake provides an instant bridge of communication. A reason to talk to people. A reason to smile. A reason to step out of my shell.

Within a couple of months of finding Jake, I was right back down to 180 pounds, and while I missed Peety every single day, I found that I could miss him and still be happy.

That's when I realized that a dog and me just go together. It's simply meant to be.

I was out on a woodsy trail, running with Jake, when I made a promise to myself that I would never be without a dog for the rest of my life. No matter what.

Peety and his unconditional love came along at just the right time. He came into my life, and simply by being there, he rescued me. He saved me. All of me. In just about every way a man can be saved.

And then, when I desperately needed to be rescued again, Jake showed up to save me, too.

There was a time in my life when I might have written that all off as some sort of coincidence, or maybe luck.

I know better now.

There are millions of dogs out there looking to be rescued. There are millions of people in the world who need to be saved.

Sometimes, when I'm out running with Jake, with the sun on my face and the wind at my back, I close my eyes and think about Peety. I see him, clear as day, jumping up into the air all excited, circling around and around by the door just waiting to get outside for a walk with me, looking up at me with the look in his eyes that reminded me, always, just how much my presence meant.

And then I think about how many other dogs are out there, waiting for someone to walk with.

Sometimes I stop to imagine how different the world would be if more of us embraced the miracle that can be experienced through the bond and unconditional love of a rescued dog.

Does anyone else ever stop and think that maybe, just maybe, God put all of these dogs here for a reason?

I can't say for sure. And look, I'm not here to try to make anyone believe in God. That's not my job. But to me, after all I've seen, and all I've experienced, the message seems perfectly clear.

Somebody up there wants us to know that none of us—no matter how messed up or alone or tired of life we think we are—not one of us ever has to walk alone.

# Afterword

About a year and a half after Peety passed away, my friends at Humane Society Silicon Valley approached me about making a short film. I had stayed in touch with Casaundra and others, and they knew what Peety had done for me. They were launching a new initiative named Mutual Rescue™—to show people that the act of rescuing an animal often rescues the person, too—and decided a short film might be a nice way to share the power of that human-animal connection.

I sat for some interviews over the course of a couple of days. The filmmakers from Advocate Creative in Chicago used a drone to capture some beautiful shots of me out running, which I thought was pretty cool. Then they went off to edit the film—into what, exactly, I wasn't sure. They hired an artist to add some renderings of me and Peety, and then one day, they put that film online—and I was absolutely blown away. The film was called *Eric & Peety, a Mutual Rescue™ Film*, and it told the story of Peety and me more beautifully than I ever expected anyone could.

This, finally, was the memorial to Peety that seemed fitting for all that he was. And I was grateful.

Then something extraordinary happened: the film went viral.

The SFGate website posted it to their Facebook page, and it quickly became their number one story. Within hours, the film was watched more than a million times. Within a month, the view count soared to over thirty million views on that site. People liked it and shared it all over the place. Other Facebook pages and websites picked it up, too. Soon, it spread across the web—and all around the world. Globally, the film has now been viewed more than one hundred million times. But it didn't stop there. The popularity of Peety's story led to all sorts of magazine articles, speaking engagements, an appearance on *The Rachael Ray Show*, and even to this book.

That six-minute film changed my life.

It changed Jake's, too. He became a celebrity as a result of the film. He's got his own fan base now. And just like Peety, he definitely loves all the attention.

It seemed like a miracle that Peety managed to touch people all over the world even though he was no longer with us. And I marvel every day at how he continues to affect my life in ways that extend beyond my wildest imagination.

Moved by Peety's story, people from all over the world have contacted me with their stories of miracle dogs in their own lives, and shared their sometimes heartbreaking stories of personal struggles with weight and health. For some, the message of our film was all about the power one dog has to love and inspire love in others. For some, it was all about the simple message of how important it is to get healthy, and the enormous power we have within each of us to change our bodies for the better. For others still, the film served as the inspiration they needed to go out and rescue a dog themselves, and to begin to transform their own lives for the better.

I was grateful for every message I received, and especially grateful for one: I received a message from Peety's previous owner—the woman who surrendered him to HSSV.

Even though his name had changed, she couldn't get over just how much the dog in that film looked like Raider, the dog she had given up for adoption. She watched it again and again—and finally, she reached out to me.

I was absolutely elated to hear from her.

I confirmed for her that Peety was, in fact, Raider. She asked me all about the stories in the film and wanted to know how Peety had lived out his final days. I told her how his last act of heroism was jumping six feet in the air to save me from an aggressive panhandler.

"Wow," she said. "Yeah. He was always super protective of my girls."

"I always wondered where the heck he learned to jump like that," I said. "Did you guys have him in Frisbee competitions or something?"

"No, nothing like that," she said. She paused for a moment. "I mean, it's not a great story, really. When we kept him in the backyard, we had this big wooden privacy fence. It must have been six feet tall. And whenever a car would come in the driveway or the mailman came walking up to the house or the kids came home, Peety would jump up and down just to see who it was. He would jump way up just to peek over the top of that fence, you know? He only saw them for half a second before he fell back down, so he would jump right back up again, over and over and over, like he was on a pogo stick or something."

"Wow," I said. "So, that must've really built up the muscles in his legs."

"Yeah," she said. She began to cry. "I just feel so bad, you know? I think he just wanted to be with another human being so much."

I pictured my Peety penned up behind that fence, and it took us both a minute to stop crying.

"Well," I finally said. "I hope you know that you did the right thing by taking him to the shelter. He was surrounded by people who loved and cared for him, right from the start. They put him in a foster program, so he was in a home and not in a cage. And then he connected with me, and I was there for him every day. And he was there for me."

I told her about some of his adventures. The road trip. The train rides. Riding to the top of the Space Needle.

"He lived a really great life these last few years," I said.

She let out a big sigh and seemed to stop crying at that point. "I'm so glad," she said. "I'm so glad to know that. You have no idea how much guilt I've carried."

"Well, no more guilt, OK? You did the right thing. I mean it. Thank you. That stuff you saw in the film, I mean, that was all true. He saved my life. Truly saved my life. That might not have happened if you didn't bring him to the shelter. So you not only helped him. You helped *me*."

Connecting with that woman, gaining answers to mysteries about Peety's prior life, allowing her to shed her deep sense of guilt—all of that was a gift I never even imagined.

And the gifts kept coming.

In the fall of 2016 I received an e-mail from someone I hadn't heard from since I was seventeen years old: Jaye, my first love, the girl who loved me just for being me way back when I was an awkward teen. She happened to see the film on the Internet one day and simply could not believe her eyes. She cried, she said. She always wondered what had happened to me, and had searched for me for quite some time. I had also been searching for her for years, hoping to one day see her again. Until she saw that film, she said, she thought I might be dead!

Jaye provided her phone number in that e-mail. "If you have any interest in reconnecting with an old friend, I'd love it if you gave me a call."

I called her the very second I read those words.

It was so good to hear her voice.

It turns out Jaye had gone through her own epic journey in life. She had two grown children now. She'd struggled through and emerged from some serious trials. It seemed as if both of us had been lost in the wilderness for the last forty years.

Talking to her was as easy and natural as it had been back when we were kids. One long phone call turned into two, then three, then four, then more. We arranged our schedules and bought airline tickets so we could see each other as soon as possible. Then, when we finally connected in person, we hugged for what felt like an eternity.

It was as if no time at all had passed between us. Sure, we

both looked a little older on the outside. But our attraction to each other was as young as ever. The spark was still there. We both wanted a forever relationship. We had both been through enough and learned enough to finally become our best selves—to emerge from shells we had long ago climbed into—and both of us were now ready to embrace the love we had to give.

In a matter of weeks, and with Jake's approval, Jaye packed her things and moved halfway across the country to move in with me. A couple of months later, we both agreed that living together simply wasn't enough. So we flew to Hawaii and got married.

After forty years of struggling to find the sort of love we were both after, it was Peety who finally brought us both home. I let him take the lead, and he led me all the way back to my very first love. The love of my life.

Even in death, Peety was still working his magic. He served as my conduit, my bridge, and my guide, and today he continues to lead me forward. I trust in him, fully. I have no reason not to. And that is why as this journey of ours continues to unfold I will follow him wherever he leads.

I know some people might think it's silly, but I am absolutely convinced of one thing: God brings angels into our lives, and angels aren't always human.

# Acknowledgments

My story would not have been possible without the help of many wonderful people who inspired me to transform from the sad, forgotten, and dying man I was to the joyous, fulfilled, and fit man I am today. In addition to the individuals named in this book, I would like to thank these people from the bottom of my heart, each of whom provided inspiration for this book and whose kindness and wisdom made me a better man:

Carol Novello, Finnegan Dowling, and Casaundra Cruz and all the staff and volunteers of Humane Society Silicon Valley, thank you for everything you do to find loving homes for homeless animals, and especially for helping Peety and everything you did to publicize our story.

· Melissa and Carlos Murillo, of San Jose, California, thank you for your selflessness in fostering surrendered animals with special needs, and especially for providing Peety a foster home until he found me.

*Acknowledgments*

Dr. Preeti Kulkarni, ND, of Core Integrative Health in Cupertino, California, thank you for saving my life by properly diagnosing the underlying cause of my medical problems and illuminating my path to health.

Timi and John Sobrato, thank you for your kindness and generosity in sponsoring the *Eric & Peety* film that led to this book. David Whitman, vice president of Mutual Rescue™, thank you for your vision in developing the concept of the film. And to the entire team at Advocate Creative in Chicago, thank you for honoring Peety with your extraordinary filmmaking and illustrating skills.

Michelle Taylor Cehn, Lindsay Dadko, and Margaret Kaye Curtis, of the San Francisco Bay Area vegan community, thank you for your friendship and for inspiring me with your courage, compassion, and kindness to animals.

Vicki Araujo, Meghan Newell, Marcia Duong, Vinh Ngo, Albert Pham, Debbie Simms, Tina Le, Cynthia Lim, and all my other friends in the Bay Area Runners, RunningAddicts, and Go Far Run Group, thank you for your friendship and for introducing me to the sport of long distance running and the glorious running trails of Northern California.

Chef Philip Gelb of Oakland, California, thank you for teaching me the culinary skills needed to prepare a complete symphony of flavorful and fragrant world cuisines from whole plants.

Lynda Nguyen-Le of San Jose, California, thank you for helping a special-needs old man through his science classes at De Anza College. I could not have passed my classes without you.

Craig Cracchiolo of GE Appliances and Mark Collier of

Whirlpool Corporation, thank you for being the most rational and humane managers I have ever worked for.

Kent Wolf, my agent, Mark Dagostino, my cowriter and literary mentor, and Karen Murgolo, my editor: God bless you all for taking a chance on me and bringing my story to life.

Howard Jacobson, PhD, host of the *Plant Yourself Podcast* and contributing author to *Whole*, by T. Colin Campbell, PhD, and *Proteinaholic*, by Garth Davis, MD, thank you for your technical advice about nutrition science.

My wife, Jaye, and my mother, Susan, thank you for your love and support.

# Advice and Recommended Resources

Were you inspired by my story? Would you like to improve your health and achieve the sort of results described in this book? If so, I encourage you to keep reading—because you can do this, and it is easier than you may think.

When I reconnected with my high school girlfriend, Jaye (now my wife), in September 2016 after forty years apart, she weighed 197 pounds and was a size 20. Eight months later, in April 2017, she weighs 121 pounds and is a size 2. So how did she lose over 70 pounds in just seven months, during the winter holidays and a ten-day honeymoon in Maui? By allowing me to coach her to do the same things I did.

Jaye says the changes in her diet and lifestyle were relatively effortless with my coaching, and what she likes even better than losing the weight is the greatest feeling of health that she has ever experienced.

I want everyone to experience that feeling! And I know it is possible because I've lived it.

It starts with a decision. It starts with a commitment to

become your best *you*. When you close your eyes and visualize the awesome person you have always wanted to be, what
does that person look like, both physically and emotionally?
Commit to become that person—right now!

Once you've committed, you're on your way. But you are
unlikely to get there without help. You need a support team.
Start by consulting with a primary care physician or licensed
naturopathic doctor. If you want results like mine, be sure
to look for a doctor who is "vegan friendly," and explain
that you want a complete physical and comprehensive blood
panel before starting a mainstream program of healthy diet
and light exercise. The purpose of the physical exam and
blood tests is to assess your current physical condition and
obtain a record that you can use to compare with your "after" results when you succeed with your program, so you will
have proof of your accomplishment and can inspire others to
achieve similar results.

In addition to acquiring complete records of your physical
stats before you begin your transformation, please also make
sure to take some "before" photos to contrast with photos
showing how amazing you'll look by comparison after you
succeed with this lifestyle change. Also, if weight loss is a
part of your overall health goal, be sure to track your weight
on a spreadsheet or notepad. I suggest doing it on the same
day each week to help keep yourself motivated and to keep
a record of your progress.

Next, commit to changing your lifestyle with a healthy
diet and light daily exercise. This is not like climbing Mount
Everest! You can lose one hundred pounds or more in a year
or less just by adopting a whole-food, plant-based, no-oil

diet (following the guidance of my recommended resources on the following pages) and by walking for half an hour, twice each day. No extreme exercise is required, and you will quickly feel happier and healthier than ever.

You may want to add one more important member to your support team, as well. After receiving a physical exam and clearance from your health care provider, consider adopting a dog from a local shelter. Be sure to give this plenty of serious thought first. A dog is a lifetime commitment and shouldn't be treated as anything less than a new member of your family. A dog will require your time and love, and you have to be prepared for the cost of dog ownership for food, supplies, and veterinary bills. Next, talk with the folks at your shelter and invest the time to find the dog that's the best match for you. Your new dog will become a key member of your support team and will become your new best friend and training partner. One more bit of advice: please adopt an adolescent or adult dog rather than a puppy—an inexperienced dog owner adopting a puppy is similar to an inexperienced parent adopting a two-year-old child. An adult dog will most likely be house trained and is likely past the phase where he or she will destroy your shoes and furniture. And, most important, an adult dog will know that you saved his or her life and will see you as the most important person on the planet for the remainder of his or her days. You're unlikely to ever experience greater unconditional love and loyalty than from a rescued dog.

Walking with a dog, rather than alone, will keep you committed to your health plan and provide an eager training partner for your twice-daily walks. The dog will force you to go outside when you otherwise may want to skip your walks. And the walks will do more than just provide the light exercise needed for your body to function properly—walking before lunch and dinner will reduce your hunger hormones so that you will be inclined to eat less and will feel satisfied sooner than you would without this exercise.

Finally, realize now that you are likely to occasionally backslide and have bad days, but promise yourself that when you do, you will get back on your plan the very next day. Nobody has ever succeeded without overcoming failures.

Each of the resources I'm about to share with you helped me to adopt the lifestyle I followed to lose my weight, and the insights I gleaned from these very same resources continue to help me maintain the same weight and health six years later. Don't wait any longer. If you watch and read these resources now and adopt a whole-food, plant-based, no-oil diet—along with a loving dog to take this journey with you—within one year, you can be the amazing person you've always wanted to be!

For more ongoing guidance and recommendations from me, also be sure to visit my website: ericandpeety.com.

# Recommended Health and Nutrition Resources

## Documentaries Available on Netflix and Amazon Prime

*Forks over Knives*: The first and greatest documentary ever produced about the imperative and benefits of a whole-food, plant-based diet.

  *https://www.netflix.com/title/70185045*

*PlantPure Nation*: From the producer and writer of *Forks over Knives*,. this documentary follows the story of people on a quest to spread the message of one of the most important health breakthroughs of all time.

  *https://www.netflix.com/title/80068073*

*Cowspiracy*: This documentary exposes the impact of animal agriculture on the environment and investigates the policies of environmental organizations on this issue.

  *https://www.netflix.com/watch/80033772*

*What the Health*: Through interviews with farmers, doctors, and other experts, this film highlights the health dangers of the profit-fueled, modern industrialized diet.
  *https://www.netflix.com/title/80174177*


## Books

*How Not to Die*: The best and most comprehensive book about how a plant-based diet will maximize your life span and reduce your risk of preventable disease, including cancer, obesity, and type 2 diabetes. Includes an easy-to-follow guide on what to eat to add years to your life.
  Greger, Michael, MD, and Stone, Gene. *How Not to Die: Discover the Foods Scientifically Proven to Prevent and Reverse Disease*. New York: Flatiron Books, 2015.

*The Starch Solution*: A complete primer on how to practice a plant-based diet. Eat the foods you love, regain your health, and lose the weight for good.
  McDougall, John A., and McDougall, Mary A. *The Starch Solution: Eat the Foods You Love, Regain Your Health, and Lose the Weight for Good!* New York: Rodale, 2012.

*Forks over Knives—The Cookbook*: An extraordinary collection of recipes, all of which can be prepared from common ingredients in thirty minutes or less, and proving that the whole-food, plant-based, oil-free lifestyle is not about what you can't eat, but what you can.

Sroufe, Del. *Forks over Knives—The Cookbook: Over 300 Recipes for Plant-Based Eating All through the Year*. New York: The Experiment, 2012.

*The Engine 2 Seven-Day Rescue Diet*: The follow-up to the best seller Engine 2 Diet series, the Seven-Day Rescue Diet is a perfect kick-starter to lower your cholesterol, drop your blood sugar and blood pressure, and help you lose weight in only seven days!

Esselstyn, Rip. *Engine 2 Seven-Day Rescue Diet: Eat Plants, Lose Weight, Save Your Health*. New York: Grand Central Life & Style, 2016.

*The Engine 2 Cookbook*: Rip and Jane Esselstyn's first fully illustrated book to help readers bring the Engine 2 lifestyle into their kitchens, with 130 plant-based recipes.

Esselstyn, Rip, and Esselstyn, Jane. *The Engine 2 Cookbook*. New York: Grand Central Life & Style, 2018.

# Animal Welfare Resources

See the original *Eric & Peety* film, learn more about Mutual Rescue, see other inspiring Mutual Rescue stories, and submit your own story at www.mutualrescue.org.

Local shelters and rescue groups need your support. Local humane societies are *not* chapters of Humane Society of the United States (HSUS). If you want to save animals in your own community, please adopt, volunteer, and give locally.

**To find a shelter near you to adopt a pet, volunteer, or support, please visit:**

MutualRescue.org
Petfinder.com
Petharbor.com
adoptapet.com

## Leadership and innovation in animal welfare:

Maddie's Fund: www.maddiesfund.org

Maddie's Fund is the leading animal welfare endowment in the country, founded by Dave Duffield (cofounder of People Soft and WorkDay) and his family to inspire the animal welfare community to work together collaboratively to save lives. In 2016, they created the Maddie Hero Award to recognize the most innovative animal welfare organizations in the country. These shelters are the winners of the 2016 Maddie Hero Award:

- St. Hubert's Animal Welfare Center, Madison, NJ: www.sthuberts.org
- Charleston Animal Society, North Charleston, SC: www.charlestonanimalsociety.org
- Muttville Senior Dog Rescue, San Francisco, CA: www.muttville.org
- Oregon Humane Society, Portland, OR: www.oregonhumane.org
- Austin Pets Alive!, Austin, TX: www.austinpetsalive.org
- Humane Society Silicon Valley, Milpitas, CA: www.hssv.org (where Peety was adopted)
- Kansas City Pet Project, Kansas City, MO: kcpetproject.org
- Pet Resource Center, Hillsborough County, Tampa, FL: www.hillsboroughcounty.org/en/residents/animals-and-pets
- San Diego Humane Society & SPCA, San Diego, CA: www.sdhumane.org

Other organizations that are doing leading-edge work to help homeless animals include:

Ally Cat Allies: www.alleycat.org
Best Friends: www.bestfriends.org
Seattle Humane: www.seattlehumane.org (where Jake was adopted)

**Organizations helping homeless animals and people:**

Pets for Vets: www.pets-for-vets.com

**National organizations that focus primarily on advocacy and legislation for animals and education for the animal welfare sector:**

Humane Society of the United States www.hsus.org
ASPCA www.aspca.org
PETA www.peta.org
Farm Sanctuary www.farmsanctuary.org

# About the Authors

Eric O'Grey is an inspirational speaker with a BS degree in finance from San Jose State University and a Juris Doctor degree from Emory University. Eric's passions include his wife, Jaye, gourmet plant-based cooking, long-distance running with his dog, Jake, and kindness to animals. More information about Eric, including his efforts to help others reverse obesity and type 2 diabetes and achieve optimal weight and health, is available on his website, ericandpeety.com.

Mark Dagostino is a multiple *New York Times* best-selling coauthor whose career has been built through the sharing of uplifting and inspirational stories. His books include titles with Chip and Joanna Gaines, Notre Dame legend Rudy Ruettiger, Villanova basketball coach Jay Wright, and professional wrestler Hulk Hogan. Before becoming an author, Mark served ten years on staff in New York and LA as a correspondent, columnist, and senior writer for *People* magazine. More information is available on his website, markdagostino.com.